Anatomy, Stretching & Training for Yoga

Anatomy, Stretching & Training for Yoga

A Step-by-Step Guide to Getting the Most from Your Yoga Practice

Amy Auman and Lisa Purcell

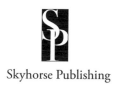

Skyhorse Publishing

Copyright © 2013 by Amy Auman and Lisa Purcell

Photos Copyright © 2010 by Jonathan Conklin Photography, Inc.

Produced for Skyhorse Publishing by Moseley Road, Inc. (www.moseleyroad.com)

Skyhorse Publishing books may be purchased in bulk at special discounts for sales promotion, corporate gifts, fund-raising, or educational purposes. Special editions can also be created to specifications. For details, contact the Special Sales Department, Skyhorse Publishing, 307 West 36th Street, 11th Floor, New York, NY 10018 or info@skyhorsepublishing.com.

Skyhorse® and Skyhorse Publishing® are registered trademarks of Skyhorse Publishing, Inc. ®, a Delaware corporation.

www.skyhorsepublishing.com

10 9 8 7 6 5 4 3 2 1

Library of Congress Cataloging-in-Publication Data is available on file.

ISBN: 978-1-62873-637-3

Printed in China

CONTENTS

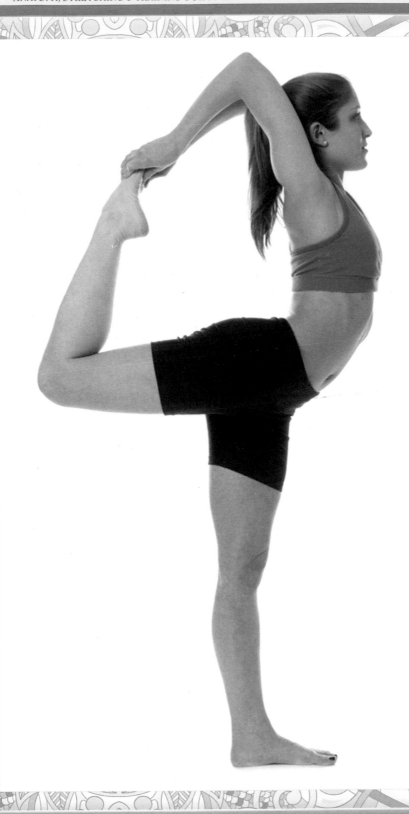

INTRODUCTION

The practice of yoga, developed in India thousands of years ago, aims to educate the body, mind, and spirit. Today, this ancient system has become one of the most popular ways of both getting fit and finding some serenity in today's hectic world. Through breathing techniques and mastering a series of poses—known as *asanas*—as a student of yoga you will truly refresh your body, mind, and spirit.

The following pages will focus on the physical aspects of yoga and feature more than fifty asanas common to many yoga disciplines. Step-by-step photos and anatomical illustrations guide you through attaining the asanas, with the visible working muscles in each asana highlighted in the illustrations. There are also handy tips that guide you as you learn to achieve and hold each asana, as well as a list of benefits, cautions, and each asana's target muscles.

A section on yoga breathing introduces you to the practice of yoga. Next you will learn a variety of asanas. The asanas are grouped into six sections—Warm-up, Resting & Rejuvenating Asanas, Standing & Balancing Asanas, Forward Bends, Yoga Backbends, Seated Asanas & Twists, and Arm Supports & Inversions. The final section of the book helps you pull the asanas you've learned into flowing sequences.

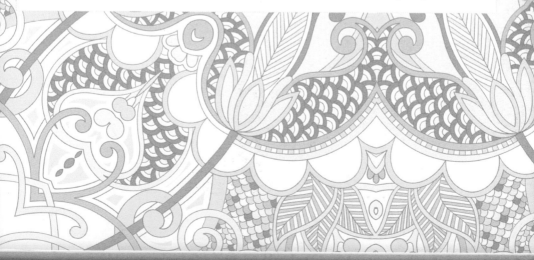

BREATHING BASICS

YOGA IS LARGELY embodied by the physical poses, or asanas, that one practices. The asanas focus on strength, flexibility, and bodily control. Beneath our structure of bones, tendons, and muscles, however, there is an entire respiratory system working simultaneously. Similar to the processes in digestion and cellular function, breathing draws nutrients into your body and expels waste.

Breath is the link between our physical and mental selves, and breath control, or Pranayama, is an important yoga practice that you should exercise separately and incorporate into the asana practice. Expanding and strengthening your breath and mind, then, coincides with stretching and strengthening your body.

Prananyama

Practicing Pranayama means to control your internal pranic energy, or breath of life. *Apana* refers to the elimination of breath—the alternate action of *prana*. While you intake the breath of life, you must also eliminate the toxins within the depths of your respiratory system.

There are numerous Pranayama exercises for you to practice the movement of *prana*. Featured here are examples of both rejuvenating and relaxing exercises; all of them will replenish fresh oxygen to your lungs and connect your mind with your body.

Samavrtti: Same Action

Observe the irregularities of your breathing, and transition into a slower and more even breath. To achieve the same action, or Samavrtti, inhale for four counts, and then exhale for four counts. This breathing technique calms the mind and creates a sense of balance and stability.

Ujjayi: The Victorious Breath

Ujjayi is sometimes called the "ocean breath" because of the sound air makes as it passes through the narrowed epiglottal passage. Maintaining the same even rhythm as the breath in Samavritti, constrict your epiglottis in the back of your throat to practice Ujjayi. Keep your mouth closed, and listen for the hiss in the back of your throat. Ujjayi breathing tones internal organs, increases internal body heat, improves concentration, and calms the mind and body.

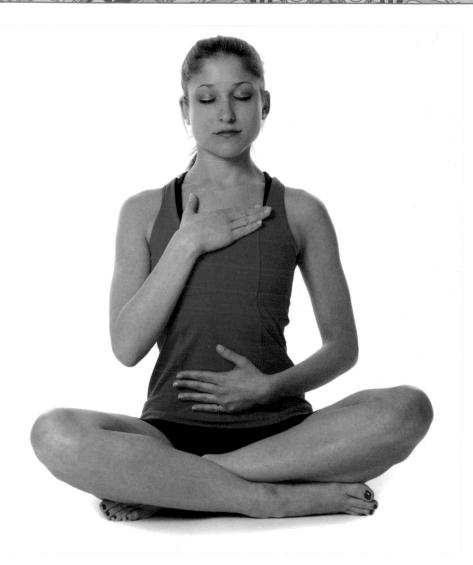

PREPARING FOR PRANAYAMA

Before practicing Pranayama in seated positions, lie down in Savasana (see page 27) to focus on your breath. Breathe evenly, and focus on filling every part of your lungs with oxygen. Air should fill your lungs from the bottom up. First, your diaphragm expands to fill your abdomen. Air then fills the middle of your lungs within your rib cage, until it finally reaches the top of your lungs, indicated by the rising of your chest. Both sides of your chest should rise equally. Most people only fill the top of their lungs with air, leaving the bottom portions largely deprived of proper nourishment. When you are ready to practice Pranayama in a comfortable seated position, begin by placing one hand on your chest and the other on your abdominals. This will help you observe your breath. Close your eyes, lift up out of your spine, tuck your chin slightly toward your sternum, and listen to your breath as your rib cage and abdominals expand and contract. Focus on the pathway your breath travels, the rhythm, and the texture of the sound.

BREATHING BASICS

Kumbhaka: Retaining the Breath

Kumbhaka is the practice of holding your breath. Begin by practicing Ujjayi or Samavrtti breathing. After every four successive breaths, hold your breath in Kumbhaka for four to eight counts. Then, allow your exhalation to last longer than your inhalation. Initially, your Kumbhaka will be shorter than your other breaths. Eventually, reduce the number of breaths in between Kumbhaka breaths and increase the number of counts in

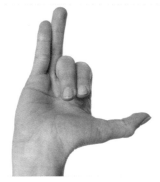

To form the Vishnu Mudra hand position, curl your index and middle fingers down, while keeping your ring finger and pinkie close together and pointed upward.

your inhale, exhale, and Kumbhaka. Build up to an exhalation twice as long as your inhalation and a Kumbhaka breath three times as long. Kumbhaka practice strengthens the diaphragm, restores energy, and cleanses the respiratory system.

Anuloma Viloma: Alternate Nostril Breathing

Anuloma Viloma purifies the energy channels, or *nadis*, through the right and left nostrils. This stimulates the movement of prana. Begin by forming the Vishnu Mudra hand position, with your index and middle fingers of your right hand curled down. Place your thumb on the outside of your right nostril, and inhale through your left nostril, keeping your mouth closed. Close your left nostril with your ring finger at the top of the breath, and

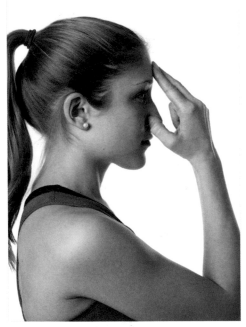

To stimulate Ajna chakra, place your index and middle fingers on your forehead. The Ajna chakra is known as the chakra of the mind. This space between your eyebrows is said to be where the nadis energy channels through your nostrils and meets with the central nadi. This is a very powerful hand position in Pranayama practice.

hold momentarily. Lift your thumb, and exhale out of your right nostril. Then, inhale with your right nostril, and so on. Begin with five cycles, gradually increasing the number of cycles with practice. Anuloma Viloma lowers the heart rate and relieves stress.

Kapalabhati: The Shining Skull

Kapalabhati breathing incorporates a rhythmic pumping action in the abdominals to exhale.

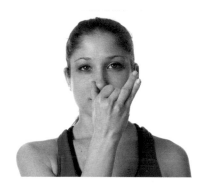

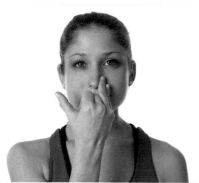

In the Vishnu Mudra hand position, close your right nostril with your right thumb, and inhale through your left. Hold your breath, squeezing both nostrils with your ring finger and your thumb, and then release your thumb to exhale through your right nostril.

Begin by loosening your abdominal muscles, and then fill your diaphragm with air. Next, push the air out of your belly in a quick, explosive exhale. The inhalation will automatically follow. This is one cycle. Begin with two rounds of ten cycles and gradually build to four rounds of twenty cycles. Kapalaphati strengthens the diaphragm, restores energy, and cleanses the respiratory system.

Sithali: The Cooling Breath

Unlike most other Pranayama exercises, inhalation occurs through the mouth in Sithali breathing. To practice Sithali, curl the sides of your tongue, and stick it slightly outside of your mouth. Inhale through the divot of your tongue. Retain your breath, close your mouth, and exhale through your nose. Continue to five or ten cycles. Sithali cools the body, providing comfort.

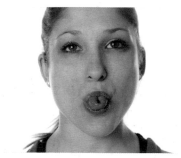

Sithali breathing literally cools your body. Curl your tongue, and inhale through your mouth.

FULL-BODY ANATOMY

FRONT

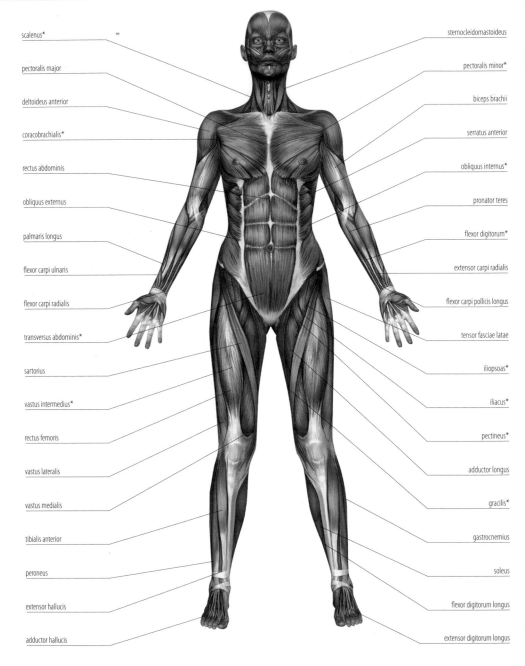

scalenus*

pectoralis major

deltoideus anterior

coracobrachialis*

rectus abdominis

obliquus externus

palmaris longus

flexor carpi ulnaris

flexor carpi radialis

transversus abdominis*

sartorius

vastus intermedius*

rectus femoris

vastus lateralis

vastus medialis

tibialis anterior

peroneus

extensor hallucis

adductor hallucis

sternocleidomastoideus

pectoralis minor*

biceps brachii

serratus anterior

obliquus internus*

pronator teres

flexor digitorum*

extensor carpi radialis

flexor carpi pollicis longus

tensor fasciae latae

iliopsoas*

iliacus*

pectineus*

adductor longus

gracilis*

gastrocnemius

soleus

flexor digitorum longus

extensor digitorum longus

ANNOTATION KEY

* indicates deep muscles

BACK

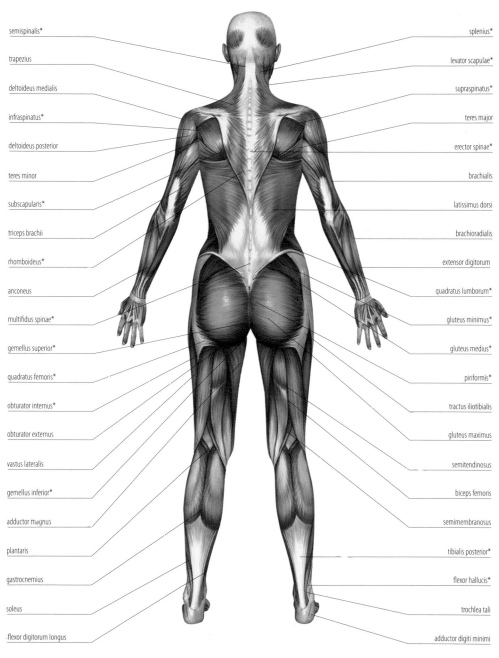

semispinalis*

trapezius

deltoideus medialis

infraspinatus*

deltoideus posterior

teres minor

subscapularis*

triceps brachii

rhomboideus*

anconeus

multifidus spinae*

gemellus superior*

quadratus femoris*

obturator internus*

obturator externus

vastus lateralis

gemellus inferior*

adductor magnus

plantaris

gastrocnemius

soleus

flexor digitorum longus

splenius*

levator scapulae*

supraspinatus*

teres major

erector spinae*

brachialis

latissimus dorsi

brachioradialis

extensor digitorum

quadratus lumborum*

gluteus minimus*

gluteus medius*

piriformis*

tractus iliotibialis

gluteus maximus

semitendinosus

biceps femoris

semimembranosus

tibialis posterior*

flexor hallucis*

trochlea tali

adductor digiti minimi

ANNOTATION KEY

* indicates deep muscles

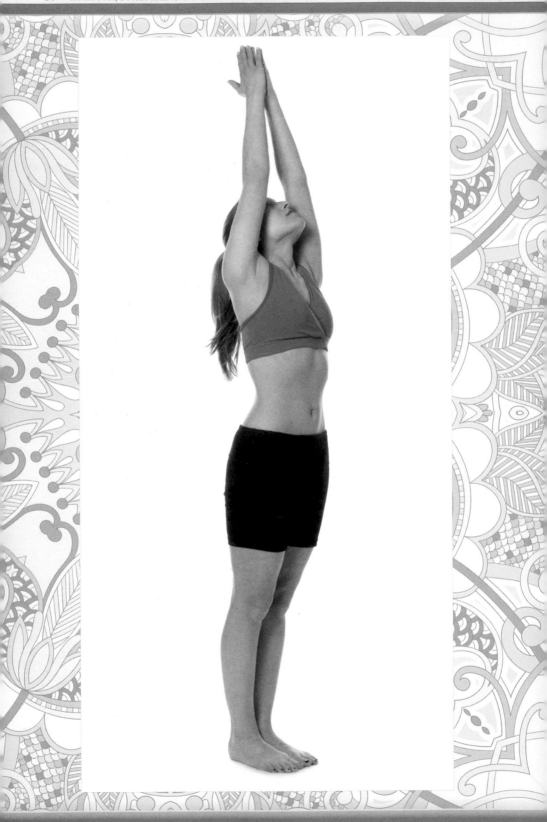

WARM-UP, RESTING & REJUVENATING ASANAS

The warm-up, resting, and rejuvenating asanas ensure that you reap all the benefits of your yoga routine. The first asanas that you practice are meant to awaken your muscles, increase your heart rate, and release tension in your body, and the last are meant to relax your muscles, lower your heart rate, and provide relief after an invigorating workout. Gentle stretching, especially after you exercise, is vital to injury prevention. In these asanas, integrate your mind, body, and breath to find the focus that you need in your yoga practice.

As well as warming you up, poses such as Sukhasana and Dandasana form the foundation of most seated postures, and forward-bending poses like Apanasana serve as counterposes to backbends. Some poses, such as Adho Mukha Svanasana, or Downward-Facing Dog, will appear in common yoga sequences, such as the Sun Salutations, so mastering them is essential for any beginner. A pose such as Balasana is a great resting pose—you can assume it in between other poses to release a tight back.

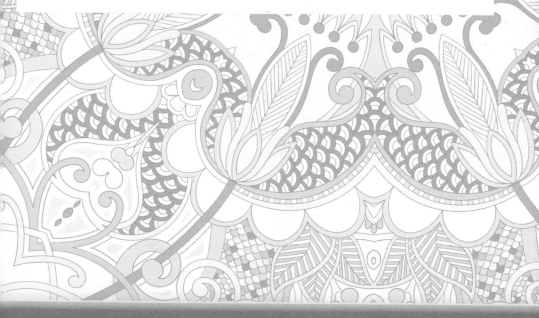

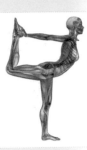

SUKHASANA

(Easy Pose; Pleasant Pose; Pose of Happiness)

SUKHASANA, OR EASY POSE, is also know as Pleasant Pose or Pose of Happiness because this relaxed position is one most of us came easily into as children. Think of how often you once sat cross-legged on the floor, content and happy. As an adult, though, you've probably spend more time in chairs than on the floor, so at first your hips and knees may feel tight. With practice, this asana will soon fit its "easy" name.

PRIMARY TARGETS
- rectus abdominis
- erector spinae
- iliopsoas
- sartorius
- transversus abdominis

BENEFITS
- Opens hips
- Strengthens spine
- Relieves stress

CAUTIONS
- Knee injury
- Hip injury

PERFECT YOUR FORM
- To help maintain neutrality in your pelvis, place the edge of a folded blanket beneath your sit bones.
- Relax the outsides of your feet on the floor.
- Avoid arching your lower back beyond its neutral spinal position.

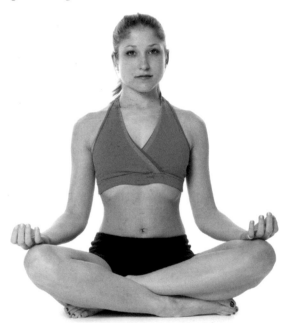

HOW TO DO IT

1 Sit on the floor with your legs extended in front of you.

2 Bend your knees, and cross your shins inward, sliding your left foot beneath your right knee and your right foot beneath your left knee, forming a gap between your feet and your groins. Relax your knees toward the floor.

3 Draw your sit bones to the floor, and lift up through your spine. Maintain a neutral position from your pelvis to your shoulders. Open your chest, and relax your shoulders.

4 Place the backs of your hands on your knees, forming an "O" with your thumb and index finger. Keep your breath slow and even.

5 Hold for as long as you wish. Be sure to also practice the pose with your opposite leg in front.

DANDASANA

(Staff Pose)

DANDASANA PROVIDES YOU with a foundation for all the seated yoga asanas, including forward bends and twists. Known as Staff Pose, this simple asana teaches you to sit with correct posture. Be sure to keep your lower body grounded while maintaining erect posture.

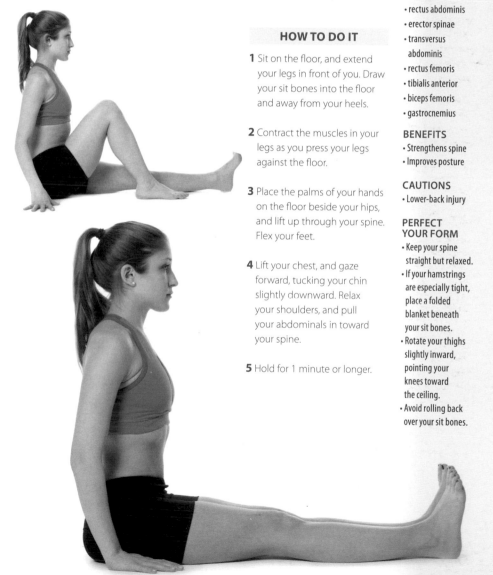

WARM-UP, RESTING & REJUVENATING ASANAS

HOW TO DO IT

1 Sit on the floor, and extend your legs in front of you. Draw your sit bones into the floor and away from your heels.

2 Contract the muscles in your legs as you press your legs against the floor.

3 Place the palms of your hands on the floor beside your hips, and lift up through your spine. Flex your feet.

4 Lift your chest, and gaze forward, tucking your chin slightly downward. Relax your shoulders, and pull your abdominals in toward your spine.

5 Hold for 1 minute or longer.

PRIMARY TARGETS
• rectus abdominis
• erector spinae
• transversus abdominis
• rectus femoris
• tibialis anterior
• biceps femoris
• gastrocnemius

BENEFITS
• Strengthens spine
• Improves posture

CAUTIONS
• Lower-back injury

PERFECT YOUR FORM
• Keep your spine straight but relaxed.
• If your hamstrings are especially tight, place a folded blanket beneath your sit bones.
• Rotate your thighs slightly inward, pointing your knees toward the ceiling.
• Avoid rolling back over your sit bones.

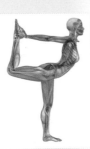

AGNISTAMBHASANA

(Fire Log Pose; Double Pigeon Pose; Knee-to-Ankle Pose; Square Pose)

LIKE LOGS STACKED in a fireplace, your shins are stacked atop each other in Agnistambhasana, or Fire Log Pose. Keep your breath steady and even during this intense hip-opening asana, in which you will certainly feel the burn.

PRIMARY TARGETS
- iliopsoas
- adductor magnus
- adductor longus
- tensor fasciae latae
- pectineus
- vastus lateralis
- vastus medialis
- gracilis
- sartorius

BENEFITS
- Stretches hips and groins

CAUTIONS
- Knee injury
- Groin injury

PERFECT YOUR FORM
- Rotate out from your hips, rather than from your knees.
- If you experience discomfort when bringing your bottom ankle below your top knee, keep your foot tucked toward your back hip and focus on the position of your top ankle.
- Don't allow your feet and ankles to cave inward.

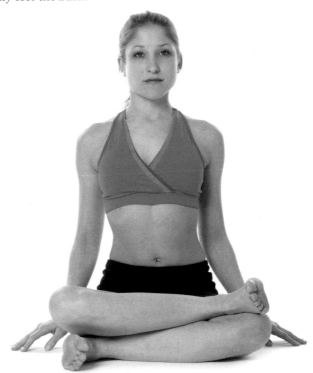

HOW TO DO IT

1 Sit in Sukhasana (see page 18) with your torso lifted tall.

2 Bend your knees and bring your legs in one at a time, placing your right ankle on top of your left knee. Your right foot should rest on the outside of your left knee.

3 Slide your left ankle below your right knee, so that your shins are stacked one on top of the other. Flex your feet.

4 Lift up in your spine through your torso to sit tall on your sit bones. Exhale, and allow your hips to open.

5 Hold for 1 to 3 minutes.

6 To come out of the pose, inhale your torso upright and uncross your legs. Repeat with your left leg on top.

VIRASANA

(Hero Pose)

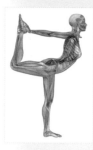

A BASIC SEATED POSTURE, Virasana, or Hero Pose, keeps your knees mobile and healthy. It is also a very calming posture and is excellent for seated meditation. A blanket or towel placed under your feet will help alleviate any discomfort you may feel on the tops of your feet.

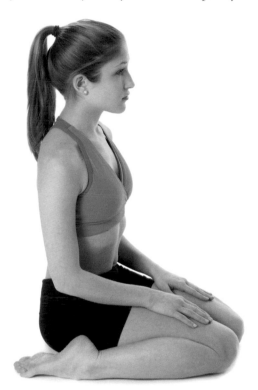

WARM-UP, RESTING & REJUVENATING ASANAS

PRIMARY TARGETS
• rectus femoris
• vastus intermedius
• tensor fasciae latae
• sartorius
• vastus medialis
• vastus lateralis
• tibialis anterior
• extensor hallucis
• peroneus

BENEFITS
• Loosens thighs, knees, and ankles
• Counterbalances hip-opening postures such as Padmasana (see page 122)
• Calms the brain for meditation
• Alleviates high blood pressure

CAUTIONS
• Knee injury
• Ankle injury

PERFECT YOUR FORM
• If you experience pain in your knees, place a folded blanket beneath you to elevate your hips. Point your big toes slightly inward so that the tops of your feet lie flat on the floor.
• Avoid turning the soles of your feet out to the sides.
• Avoid sitting on top of your heels.

HOW TO DO IT

1 Kneel on your hands and knees on the floor. Your thighs should be perpendicular to the floor, and your feet should be angled slightly wider than your hips.

2 Bring your knees together until they touch, pushing the tops of your feet into the floor. Lean forward slightly with your torso, exhaling, and begin to sit back onto your buttocks.

3 Sit on the floor with your buttocks in between your heels.

4 Lift your chest, and press your shoulders back and down, lengthening your tailbone into the floor so that you are resting on your sit bones. Place your hands on the tops of your thighs. Pull your abdominals in toward your spine.

5 Hold for 30 seconds to 1 minute.

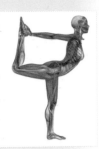

ADHO MUKHA SVANASANA

(Downward-Facing Dog; Down Dog)

PERFORMED AS A PART of the Sun Salutations, Adho Mukha Svanasana, or Downward-Facing Dog, is both an inversion and an arm balance. It provides a resting point in the yoga flows, while stretching both your back and shoulders.

PRIMARY TARGETS

- gluteus maximus
- latissimus dorsi
- semitendinosus
- semimembranosus
- biceps femoris
- rectus femoris
- gastrocnemius
- triceps brachii
- deltoideus posterior
- serratus anterior

BENEFITS

- Stretches calves, shoulders, and hamstrings
- Strengthens arms and legs
- Relieves stress and headaches

CAUTIONS

- Carpal tunnel syndrome

PERFECT YOUR FORM

- If your hamstrings and shoulders are tight, practice the pose with your knees slightly bent and your heels lifted from the floor.
- Contract your thighs to lengthen your spine further and keep pressure off your shoulders.
- Avoid sinking your shoulders into your armpits, creating an arch in your back.

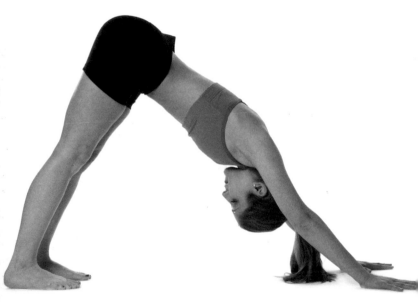

HOW TO DO IT

1 Kneel on your hands and knees with your knees directly below your hips. Stretch your hands out slightly in front of your shoulders with your fingertips facing forward. They should be placed one shoulder-width apart.

2 Exhale and press against the floor, keeping your elbows straight. Lift your sit bones up toward the ceiling and your knees away from the floor. Lengthen your hips away from your ribs to elongate your spine.

3 Press your heels toward the floor, and contract your thighs. Try to straighten your knees. Turn your thighs slightly inward, and broaden your chest and shoulders. Position your head in between your arms.

4 Hold for 30 seconds to 2 minutes.

UTTANA SHISHOSANA

(Extended Puppy Pose)

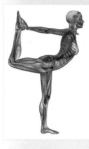

A SIMPLE FORWARD BEND, Uttana Shishosana, or Extended Puppy Pose, is an effective warm-up that makes a great follow-up to Downward-Facing Dog. It also works as a cooldown pose to relax the mind and body to relieve stress.

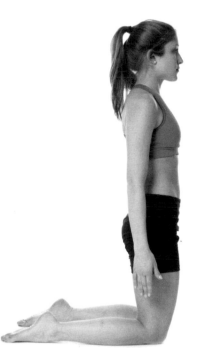

HOW TO DO IT

1 Kneel with your knees directly below your hips. Your fingertips should be facing forward with your hands one shoulder-width apart.

2 Bend forward until you are on your hands and knees, with your wrists directly below your shoulders.

3 Exhale, and press your hips back while lowering your chest toward the floor. Keep your elbows straight and lifted off the floor.

4 Relax your forehead on the floor. Stretch forward through your arms and back through your sit bones to deepen the stretch through your spine.

5 Hold for 30 seconds to 1 minute.

PRIMARY TARGETS

- gluteus maximus
- latissimus dorsi
- triceps brachii
- deltoideus posterior
- serratus anterior

BENEFITS

- Stretches the shoulders and spine

CAUTIONS

- Knee injury

PERFECT YOUR FORM

- Slightly arch your upper back, providing your shoulders and spine with a gentle and stress-relieving stretch.
- Aim to stretch your spine in both directions to get the most from this pose.
- Avoid resting your elbows on the floor.
- Avoid allowing your torso to sink at the middle.
- Don't release too quickly from the pose—as with any inverted pose, fast-changing blood flow can cause dizziness.

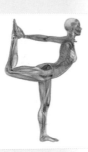

URDHVA HASTASANA

(Upward Salute; Upward Hand Pose; Raised Hands Pose)

URDHVA HASTASANA IS A NATURAL wake-up stretch that invigorates you from fingertips to toes. This basic standing asana may be easy to master, but it has the added benefit of preparing you for more advanced arm balances and backbends.

PRIMARY TARGETS
- obliquus externus
- obliquus internus
- transversus abdominis
- latissimus dorsi
- teres major
- infraspinatus
- serratus anterior
- deltoideus posterior
- biceps brachii
- triceps brachii

BENEFITS
- Fights fatigue
- Stretches abdominals, shoulders, and armpits
- Alleviates backache
- Relieves indigestion

CAUTIONS
- Shoulder injury
- Neck injury

PERFECT YOUR FORM
- Keep your shoulders aligned directly over your hips and your hips over your heels.
- Keep back ribs broad.
- Broaden the top of your shoulder blades.
- Move your armpits down while lifting the arms upward.
- Avoid jutting out your rib cage.

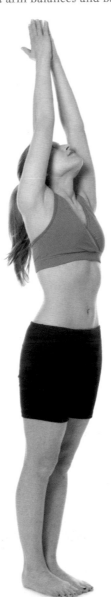

HOW TO DO IT

1 Stand in Tadasana (see pages 30–31), with your feet shoulder-width apart and your pelvis, head, and chest aligned. Turn your palms inward.

2 Keeping your arms parallel and your palms facing each other, inhale, and sweep your arms out in front of you to the height of your shoulders and then raise them upward toward the ceiling until your upper arms rest alongside your ears.

3 Spread your shoulder blades and draw your chin in slightly, as you gently tip your head back. Gaze at your thumbs.

4 Hold for 30 seconds to 1 minute.

5 Exhale, pulling your hands down with your palms together. As your hands lower toward your face, gently drop your head to a neutral position.

BALASANA

(Child's Pose)

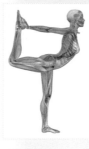

BALASANA, OR CHILD'S POSE, works wonders as a cooldown and recovery pose that stretches and releases the spine and lower back. It also works as a warm-up for forward bends or a counterpose for backbends. Balasana will leave you with a deep sense of physical, emotional, mental, and spiritual rejuvenation.

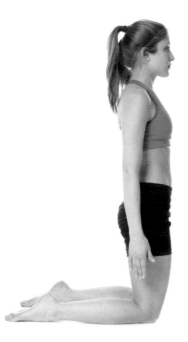

HOW TO DO IT

1 Kneel on the floor, with your hips aligned over your knees.

2 Bring your legs together so that your big toes are touching. Lower your body to rest your buttocks on your heels, and separate your knees about one hip-width apart.

3 Exhale, and lower your torso down to your inner thighs. Elongate your neck and your spine, stretching your tailbone down toward the floor.

4 Place the backs of your hands on the floor beside your feet. Allow your shoulders to relax toward the floor, widening them across your upper back. Place your forehead on the floor.

5 Hold 30 seconds to 3 minutes.

PRIMARY TARGETS
- trapezius
- latissimus dorsi
- teres major
- deltoideus posterior
- erector spinae
- gluteus maximus
- serratus anterior
- extensor digitorum longus
- tibialis anterior
- peroneus
- semitendinosus
- biceps femoris
- semimembranosus

BENEFITS
- Stretches spine, hips, thighs, and ankles
- Relieves stress

CAUTIONS
- Diarrhea
- Knee injury
- Pregnancy

PERFECT YOUR FORM
- Inhale into the back of your rib cage.
- Round your back to create a dome shape.
- Avoid compressing the back of your neck.

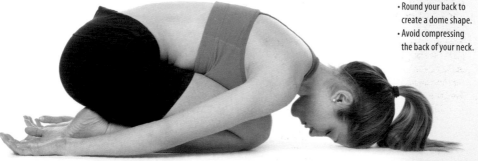

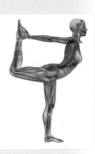

APANASANA

(Knees-to-Chest Pose; Energy-Freeing Pose; Wind-Relieving Pose)

AN EASY POSE TO EXECUTE, Apanasana, or Knees-to-Chest Pose, warms you up at the beginning of your practice and relaxes you when you are done. It releases any tension in your back or hamstrings, and can give you quick relief after a day spent sitting at a desk, or in a car, or airplane. In some yoga traditions, this pose is called Pavanmuktasana, which means "wind-relieving pose," because it helps release trapped gases from the gastrointestinal tract.

PRIMARY TARGETS
- erector spinae
- latissimus dorsi
- gluteus maximus
- gluteus minimus
- piriformis
- gemellus superior
- gemellus inferior
- obturator externus
- obturator internus
- quadratus femoris

BENEFITS
- Stretches lower back and hips
- Stimulates digestion

CAUTIONS
- Knee injury
- Pregnancy

PERFECT YOUR FORM
- Keep your spine in a neutral position.
- If you can't grasp your elbows while hugging your knees, place your hands directly on your knees instead.
- Lengthen the back of your neck.
- Avoid tensing your back or leg muscles.

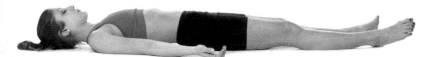

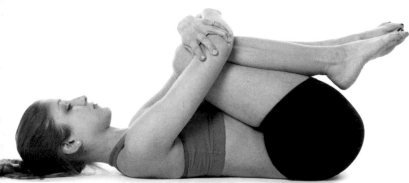

HOW TO DO IT

1 Lie supine on the floor.

2 Exhale, and draw your knees toward your chest.

3 Wrap your arms around your knees, placing each hand on your opposite elbow. Lengthen the back of your neck away from your shoulders. With each exhalation, gently pull your knees closer toward your chest, and flatten your back and shoulders on the floor.

4 Hold for 30 seconds to 1 minute.

SAVASANA

(Corpse Pose; Relaxation Pose)

MOST YOGA PRACTICE ENDS with Savasana—or Corpse Pose. When done properly, Savasana provides full-body relaxation while calming the mind. It looks easy, but mastering this asana takes time. You must learn to fully relax and let go, allowing any distractions or agitations to float past you until you achieve a deep, meditative state of rest.

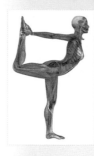

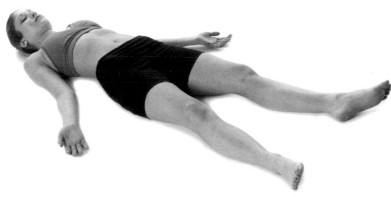

PRIMARY TARGETS
• Whole-body relaxation

BENEFITS
• Calms the brain
• Relieves stress
• Relaxes the body

CAUTIONS
• Back injury

PERFECT YOUR FORM
• End your yoga practice with Savasana.
• Pay attention to the alignment of your head, making sure that it is pulled away from your shoulders and does not tilt to one side.
• Practice with your knees bent and feet flat on the floor.
• Don't move once your body is aligned.
• Avoid tensing your muscles.

HOW TO DO IT

1 Sit on the floor with your knees bent. Lift your hips, and place your tailbone slightly closer to your heels. Elongate your lower back away from your tailbone before allowing your back to relax to the floor.

2 Straighten your legs one at a time. Allow your legs to fall open, separated the same distance from the center of your body. Your feet should be turned out equally.

3 Relax your arms on the floor by your sides, leaving a space between your torso and your arms. Spread your shoulder blades and your collarbones, and turn your arms out so that your palms face up.

4 Lengthen your neck away from your shoulders, and try to release it comfortably toward the floor. Close your eyes. Breathe smoothly. Focus on your body alignment and your breath.

5 Relax every part of your body, starting with your toes and ending with your head. Feel each part sinking into the floor. Relax the muscles in your face and calm your brain.

6 Hold for 5 to 10 minutes. Gently come out of the pose by bending your knees to your chest and rolling over to one side. Bring your head up last.

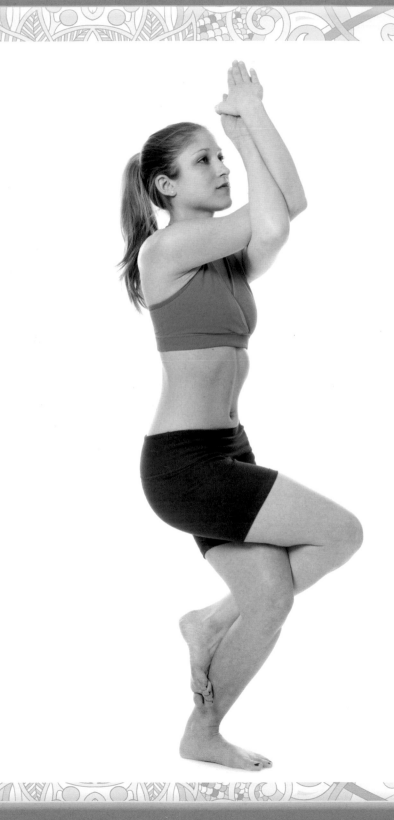

STANDING & BALANCING ASANAS

Standing asanas, generally performed at the beginning of yoga practice, build awareness of the fundamental movements of yoga. They energize your body, develop stamina, and revitalize your legs. Because they require strength, flexibility, and balance, standing asanas give insight to what areas of your body are weak or unstable. When practicing the poses in this section, be aware of your body's alignment while you find a graceful balance. It is important that you ground your feet firmly and maintain good posture.

With such a wide range of movements performed in any standing series, you will stretch and increase mobility throughout your entire body. Standing and balancing poses will strengthen your arms, shoulders, torso, pelvis, legs, and feet. Your pelvis is the link between your torso and legs, and learning to stabilize your pelvis is key to mastering standing balances. This prepares you for other asanas, such as sitting poses and arm balances.

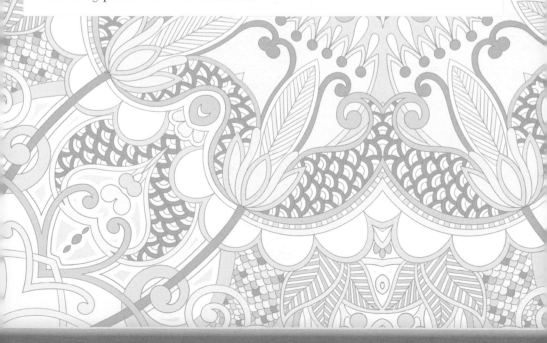

TADASANA

(Mountain Pose)

TADASANA, OR MOUNTAIN POSE, is the foundation asana that you will return to many times during your yoga practice. Tadasana may look easy—as if you are simply standing—but when done correctly, you will be as strong and unwavering as a mountain, stabilizing both your body and your mind.

ANNOTATION KEY
Black text indicates strengthening muscles
Gray text indicates stretching muscles
- - - - indicates deep muscles

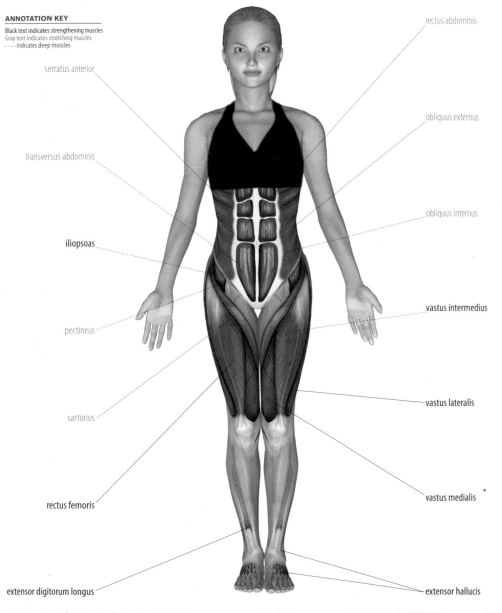

serratus anterior

transversus abdominis

iliopsoas

pectineus

sartorius

rectus femoris

extensor digitorum longus

rectus abdominis

obliquus externus

obliquus internus

vastus intermedius

vastus lateralis

vastus medialis

extensor hallucis

HOW TO DO IT

1 Stand with your feet together, with both heels and toes touching.

2 Keeping your back straight and both arms pressed slightly against your sides, face your palms outward.

3 Lift all your toes and let them fan out, and then gently drop them down to create a wide, solid base.

4 Rock from side to side until you gradually bring your weight evenly onto all four corners of both feet.

5 While balancing your weight evenly on both feet, slightly contract the muscles in your knees and thighs, rotating both thighs inward to create a widening of the sit bones.

6 Tighten your abdominals, drawing them in slightly, maintaining a firm posture.

7 Widen your collarbones, making sure your shoulders are parallel to your pelvis.

8 Lengthen your neck, so that the crown of your head rises toward the ceiling and your shoulder blades slide down your back.

9 Hold for 30 seconds to 1 minute.

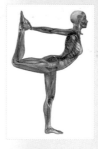

PRIMARY TARGETS

- rectus femoris
- vastus lateralis
- vastus medialis
- vastus intermedius
- iliopsoas
- piriformis
- abductor digiti minimi
- flexor hallucis
- flexor digitorum longus
- abductor hallucis
- plantar aponeurosis

BENEFITS

- Improves posture
- Strengthens thighs

CAUTIONS

- Headache
- Insomnia
- Low blood pressure

PERFECT YOUR FORM

- If your ankles are knocking together uncomfortably, slightly separate your heels.
- If you are new to yoga, practice the pose with your back to the wall to feel the alignment.
- Avoid slumping .
- Avoid drooping your shoulders.

Samasthiti, or Prayer Pose, is a variation of Tadasana. To assume Samasthiti, follow directions for Tadasana, but instead of extending your arms and fingers downward, bring your hands together at the middle of your chest, as if you were praying. Release any tension from your neck and shoulders, and then gently close your eyes. Hold the pose for 30 seconds to 1 minute.

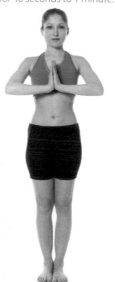

VRKSASANA

BEGINNER

(Tree Pose)

VRKSASANA CALLS FOR YOU to firmly root yourself to the ground, just as if you were a supple tree. To maintain your balance, concentrate on keeping the centerline of your body straight and steady. One of the few yoga asanas best done with eyes open, the Tree Pose will bring equilibrium to your mind and rejuvenate your body.

ANNOTATION KEY
Black text indicates strengthening muscles
Gray text indicates stretching muscles
----indicates deep muscles

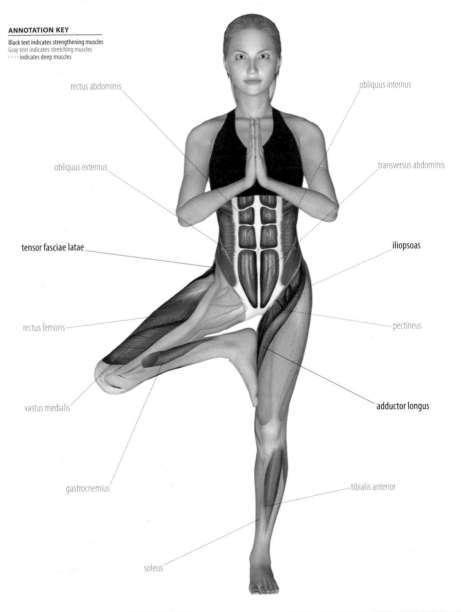

rectus abdominis

obliquus internus

obliquus externus

transversus abdominis

tensor fasciae latae

iliopsoas

rectus femoris

pectineus

vastus medialis

adductor longus

gastrocnemius

tibialis anterior

soleus

HOW TO DO IT

1 Stand in Samasthiti (see page 31). Shift your weight slightly onto your left foot, keeping your inner foot firmly grounded.

2 Bend your right knee, and reach down with your right hand and grasp your right ankle.

3 Draw your right foot up, and place the sole against your inner left thigh. Press your right heel into your inner left groin, pointing your toes toward the floor. The center of your pelvis should be directly over your left foot.

4 Rest your hands on the top rim of your pelvis. Make sure your pelvis is in a neutral position, with the top rim parallel to the floor.

5 Lengthen your tailbone toward the floor. Firmly press the sole of your right foot against your inner thigh while resisting with your outer left leg. Press your hands together, and gaze at a fixed point in front of you on the floor about 4 to 5 feet away.

6 Hold for 30 seconds to 1 minute. Exhale, and step back into Samasthiti. Repeat with your opposite leg standing.

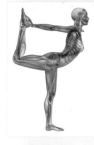

PRIMARY TARGETS

• iliopsoas
• gluteus maximus
• gluteus medius
• piriformis
• adductor magnus
• obturator internus
• obturator externus
• tensor fasciae latae
• rectus femoris

BENEFITS

• Strengthens thighs, calves, ankles, and spine
• Stretches groins, inner thighs, chest, and shoulders
• Improves sense of balance
• Relieves sciatica
• Reduces flat feet

CAUTIONS

• Headache
• Insomnia
• High or low blood pressure

PERFECT YOUR FORM

• If you are a beginner, brace your back against a wall to steady yourself.
• To keep your raised foot from sliding, place a folded sticky mat between your sole and inner thigh.
• Avoid jutting out your hip; keep both hips squared forward.

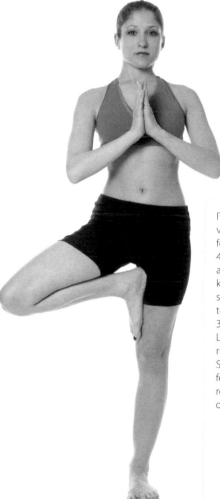

For a more advanced version of Vrksasana, follow steps 1 through 4, and then raise both arms over your head, keeping your elbows straight. Join your palms together, and hold for 30 seconds to 1 minute. Lower your arms and right leg and return to Samasthiti. Pause for a few moments, and repeat on the opposite leg.

UTKATASANA

BEGINNER *(Chair Pose; Awkward Pose; Fierce Pose; Lightning Bolt Pose; Wild Pose)*

PRACTICING UTKATASANA will increase your strength, balance, and stability while activating just about every muscle in your body. Known alternatively as Chair Pose, Awkward Pose, Fierce Pose, Lightning Bolt Pose, or Wild Pose, this asana calls for you to sustain an unsupported sitting position, which will build your stamina.

ANNOTATION KEY
Black text indicates strengthening muscles
Gray text indicates stretching muscles
----indicates deep muscles

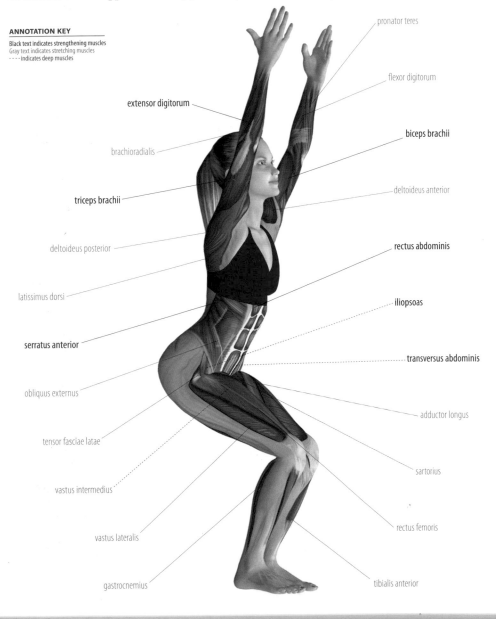

pronator teres

flexor digitorum

extensor digitorum

brachioradialis

biceps brachii

triceps brachii

deltoideus anterior

deltoideus posterior

rectus abdominis

latissimus dorsi

iliopsoas

serratus anterior

transversus abdominis

obliquus externus

adductor longus

tensor fasciae latae

sartorius

vastus intermedius

rectus femoris

vastus lateralis

tibialis anterior

gastrocnemius

HOW TO DO IT

1 Stand in Tadasana (see pages 30–31). Inhale, and raise both your hands over your head, keeping your arms straight and lengthening your spine. You may clasp your hands together or keep them shoulder-width apart.

2 Exhale, and bend your knees. Bend your upper body forward so that it is at a 45-degree angle to the floor, keeping your lower back straight. Relax your calf muscles, allowing the weight of your upper body to sink into your pelvis. Transfer your weight to your heels.

3 Hold for 30 seconds to 1 minute.

4 Inhale, and straighten your knees, lifting strongly through your arms. Exhale, release your arms to your side, and return to Tadasana.

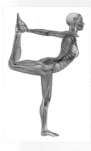

PRIMARY TARGETS
- erector spinae
- extensor digitorum
- triceps brachii
- deltoideus anterior
- deltoideus posterior
- infraspinatus
- teres major
- gluteus medius
- biceps femoris
- semitendinosus
- semimembranosus
- soleus
- tibialis anterior
- rectus femoris
- vastus lateralis
- vastus medialis
- vastus intermedius

BENEFITS
- Strengthens lower back and quadriceps
- Stretches chest, shoulders, arms, and hamstrings
- Relieves stress and tension
- Reduces flat feet

CAUTIONS
- Diarrhea
- Headache

PERFECT YOUR FORM
- Perform the lowering motion with your thighs, knees, and hips alone to achieve the proper position in your lower body.
- Avoid arching your back.

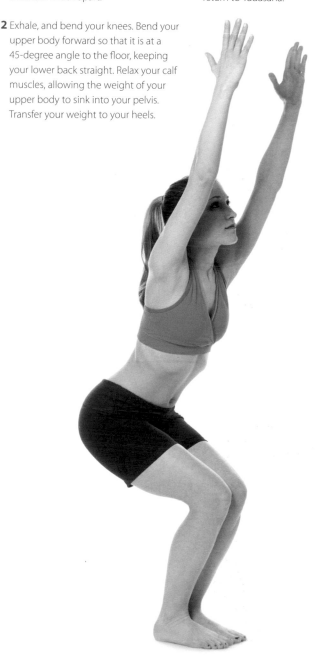

PARIVRTTA UTKATASANA

BEGINNER

(Twisting Chair Pose; Revolved Chair Pose; Prayer Twist)

BOTH A BALANCING and a twisting pose, Parivrtta Utkatasana uses just about every muscle in your body, but particularly works to strengthen your thighs, glutes, and hips. It takes the Utkatasana, or Chair Pose, a step further, challenging your sense of balance while stretching your spine, shoulders, and chest.

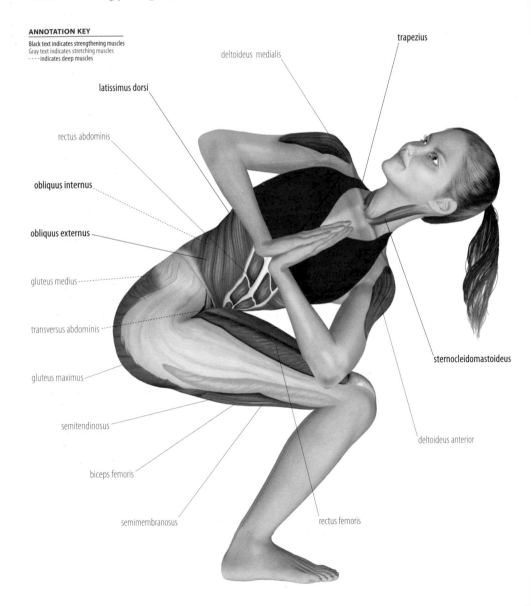

ANNOTATION KEY
Black text indicates strengthening muscles
Gray text indicates stretching muscles
- - - - indicates deep muscles

trapezius

deltoideus medialis

latissimus dorsi

rectus abdominis

obliquus internus

obliquus externus

gluteus medius

transversus abdominis

gluteus maximus

semitendinosus

biceps femoris

semimembranosus

sternocleidomastoideus

deltoideus anterior

rectus femoris

HOW TO DO IT

1 Stand in Tadasana (see pages 30–31), and then squat down in Utkatasana (see pages 34–35), with your arms extended up toward the ceiling. Lean back slightly, so that your weight rests on your heels.

2 Squeezing your legs together, inhale, and bring your hands down to your chest. Press your palms together in prayer position.

3 Exhale, and twist toward the right, lengthening your spine as you remain in the squatting position. Rotate through your spine, torso, and shoulders, and place your left elbow on the outside of your right thigh. Look up toward the ceiling.

4 With each exhalation, deepen the twist, using your left elbow to guide your rotation.

5 Hold for 10 to 30 seconds. Inhale as you untwist, returning to Tadasana before twisting to the other side.

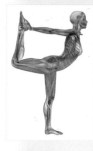

PRIMARY TARGETS
- rectus abdominis
- obliquus internus
- transversus abdominis
- biceps femoris
- rectus femoris
- obliquus externus
- gluteus medius
- gluteus maximus

BENEFITS
- Stimulates digestion
- Stretches spine
- Strengthens thighs, buttocks, and abdominals

CAUTIONS
- Back injury

PERFECT YOUR FORM
- Pull your abdominals in toward your spine, but don't tense your muscles, which will keep you from fully twisting.
- Avoid coming up from your squatted position as you twist.
- Avoid forcing a deep twist too aggressively with your elbow.

MALASANA

(Relieving Pose; Garland Pose)

MALASANA, OFTEN TRANSLATED as "Garland Pose," actually takes its name from the squatting position used to relieve oneself. It is an effective hip-opening balancing pose that also helps strengthen your thigh muscles and the muscles of your core.

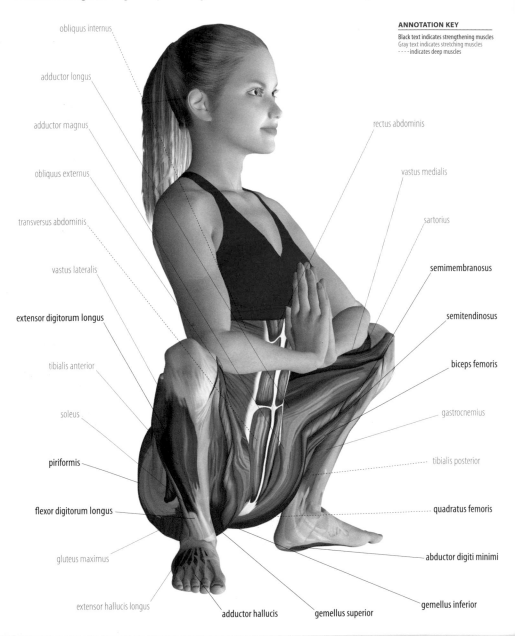

ANNOTATION KEY

Black text indicates strengthening muscles
Gray text indicates stretching muscles
----indicates deep muscles

obliquus internus

adductor longus

adductor magnus

obliquus externus

transversus abdominis

vastus lateralis

extensor digitorum longus

tibialis anterior

soleus

piriformis

flexor digitorum longus

gluteus maximus

extensor hallucis longus

adductor hallucis

rectus abdominis

vastus medialis

sartorius

semimembranosus

semitendinosus

biceps femoris

gastrocnemius

tibialis posterior

quadratus femoris

abductor digiti minimi

gemellus inferior

gemellus superior

HOW TO DO IT

1 Stand in Tadasana (see pages 30–31), with feet shoulder-width apart and your pelvis, head, and chest aligned.

2 Keeping your heels on the floor, extend your arms straight out in front of you.

3 Bend your knees, folding your body forward and down by dropping your pelvis.

4 Slightly separate your thighs wider than your torso. Exhale, and lean your body forward, fitting it snugly in the space between your thighs.

5 Press your elbows against the back of your knees, and join your palms together, as if in prayer, and then press your knees into your elbows.

6 Hold for 30 seconds to 1 minute. Exhale, and straighten your knees, slowly rising back to a standing position.

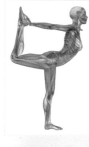

PRIMARY TARGETS
• quadratus femoris
• transversus abdominis
• biceps femoris
• sartorius
• vastus intermedius
• vastus medialis
• vastus lateralis
• semitendinosus
• semimembranosus

BENEFITS
• Stretches ankles, groins, lower legs, and back torso
• Tones abdominal and pelvic-floor muscles

CAUTIONS
• Headache
• Insomnia
• Low blood pressure

PERFECT YOUR FORM
• If your heels come up as you squat, place a folded blanket under them.
• Avoid leaning forward.
• Avoid drooping your shoulders.

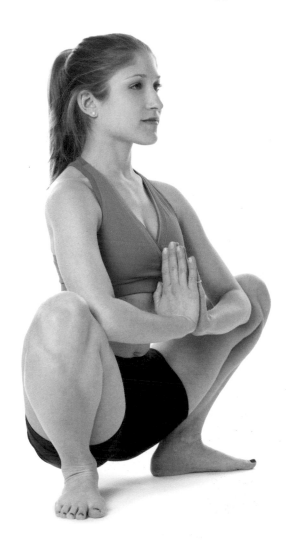

GARUDASANA

(Eagle Pose)

THIS BASIC STANDING ASANA packs a lot into a simple move: it improves your balance; stretches your upper back, shoulders, and outer thighs; and strengthens your legs, knees, and ankles. To execute Garudasana properly, you must focus equally on your upper and lower body while keeping your gaze on a point in the middle distance in front of you.

ANNOTATION KEY
Black text indicates strengthening muscles
Gray text indicates stretching muscles
- - - - indicates deep muscles

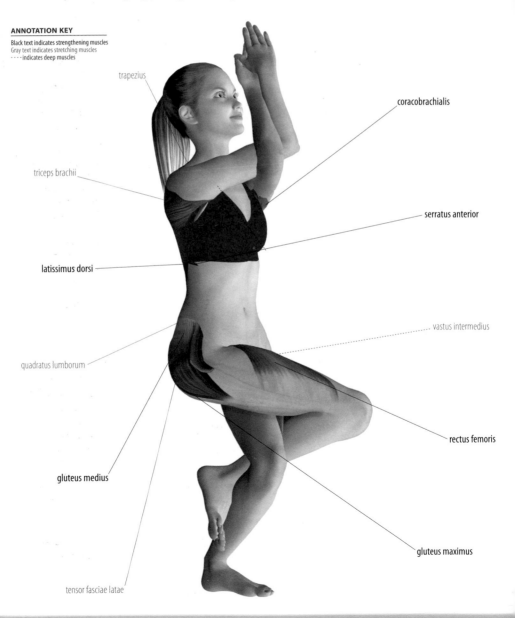

trapezius

coracobrachialis

triceps brachii

serratus anterior

latissimus dorsi

vastus intermedius

quadratus lumborum

rectus femoris

gluteus medius

gluteus maximus

tensor fasciae latae

HOW TO DO IT

1 Stand in Tadasana (see pages 30–31), with your feet shoulder-width apart and your pelvis, head, and chest aligned.

2 Shift your weight to your right leg, and then bend your knees slightly. Lift your left foot as you balance on your right foot, and cross your left thigh over the right.

3 Point your left toes toward the floor, press your foot back, and then hook the top of your foot behind your lower right calf. Maintain your balance on your right foot.

4 Inhale, and stretch your arms straight forward, keeping them parallel to the floor, and spread your scapulas wide across your back. Cross your arms in front of your torso so that your right arm is above the left, and then bend your elbows. Bring your right elbow into the crook of your left, and raise your forearms so that they are perpendicular to the floor. The backs of your hands should be facing each other.

5 Press your right hand to the right and your left hand to the left, so that your palms face each other. Your right-hand thumb should pass in front of the little finger of your left hand. Press your palms together, lift your elbows up, and stretch your fingers toward the ceiling.

6 Hold for 15 seconds to 1 minute.

7 Slowly unwind your legs and arms, and return to Tadasana. Repeat with your arms and legs reversed.

To challenge yourself, try this variation of Garudasana: Follow steps 1 through 5, and then sink down on your standing foot, bending both knees as you move downward. Bend forward from your hips, with your head facing your crossed arms. Hold for 15 seconds to 1 minute.

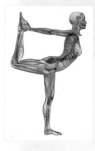

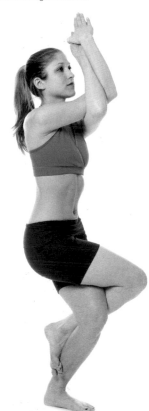

PRIMARY TARGETS
• trapezius
• infraspinatus
• teres major
• teres minor
• latissimus dorsi
• gluteus medius
• adductor magnus
• quadratus lumborum
• serratus anterior

BENEFITS
• Strengthens ankles and calves
• Stretches ankles, calves, thighs, hips, shoulders, and upper back
• Improves concentration
• Improves sense of balance

CAUTIONS
• Arm injury
• Hip injury
• Knee injury

PERFECT YOUR FORM
• If you find it difficult to wrap your arms around each other until your palms touch, stretch your arms straight forward, parallel to the floor, while holding onto the ends of a strap.
• Keep your hips squared to the front of your mat.

TRIKONASANA

BEGINNER

(Triangle Pose)

TRIKONASANA, OR TRIANGLE POSE, not only strengthens your core and legs but also stretches your torso and mobilizes your hips. It's a great beginner's pose, allowing you to improve the flexibility of both the lower and upper halves of your body. To properly maintain your balance during Trikonasana, you must keep your eyes open.

ANNOTATION KEY
Black text indicates strengthening muscles
Gray text indicates stretching muscles
----indicates deep muscles

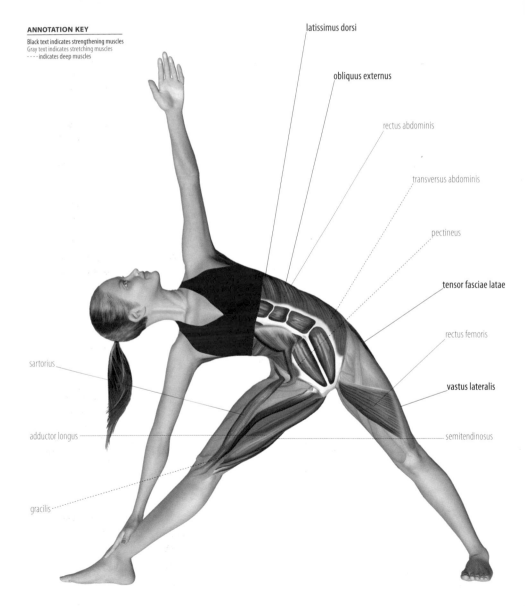

latissimus dorsi

obliquus externus

rectus abdominis

transversus abdominis

pectineus

tensor fasciae latae

rectus femoris

vastus lateralis

semitendinosus

sartorius

adductor longus

gracilis

HOW TO DO IT

1 Stand in Tadasana (see pages 30–31), with your pelvis, head, and chest aligned. Separate your feet slightly farther than the width of your shoulders.

2 Inhale, and raise both arms straight out to the side, keeping them parallel to the floor with your palms facing down.

3 Exhale slowly, and without bending your knees, pivot on your heels to turn your right foot all the way to the right and your left foot slightly toward the right, keeping your heels in line.

4 Drop your torso as far as is comfortable to the right side, keeping your arms parallel to the floor.

5 Once your torso is fully extended to the right, drop your right arm so that your right hand rests on your shin or on the front of your ankle. At the same time, extend your left arm straight up toward the ceiling. Gently twist your spine and torso counterclockwise, using your extended arms as a lever, while your spinal axis remains parallel to the ground. Extend your arms apart from each other in opposite directions.

6 Turn your head to gaze at your left thumb, intensifying the twist in your spine. Hold for 30 seconds to 1 minute.

7 Inhale, and return to a standing position with arms outstretched, strongly pressing your back heel into the floor. Reverse your feet, and repeat on the other side.

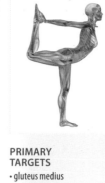

PRIMARY TARGETS
- gluteus medius
- tensor fasciae latae
- sartorius
- piriformis
- serratus anterior
- obliquus externus
- latissimus dorsi

BENEFITS
- Stretches thighs, knees, ankles, hips, groins, hamstrings, calves, shoulders, chest, and spine
- Relieves stress
- Stimulates digestion
- Relieves the symptoms of menopause
- Relieves backache

CAUTIONS
- Diarrhea
- Headache
- High or low blood pressure
- Neck issues

PERFECT YOUR FORM
- Keep your leading knee tight and aligned with the center of your leading foot, shin, and thigh.
- If you feel unsteady, brace your back heel against a wall.
- Avoid twisting from your hips.

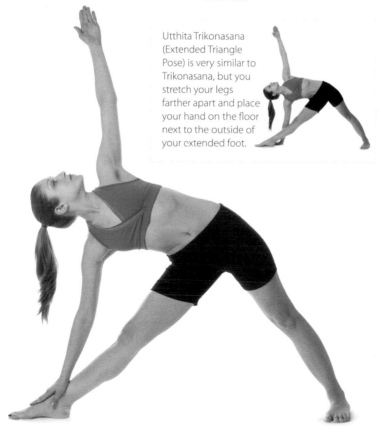

Utthita Trikonasana (Extended Triangle Pose) is very similar to Trikonasana, but you stretch your legs farther apart and place your hand on the floor next to the outside of your extended foot.

UTTHITA PARSVAKONASANA

BEGINNER

(Extended Side Angle Pose)

UTTHITA PARSVAKONASANA IS ANOTHER great pose for yoga novices who want to slowly learn how to properly stretch and contort their bodies in preparation for more advanced asanas. It also simultaneously strengthens your legs, core, and upper torso.

ANNOTATION KEY

Black text indicates strengthening muscles
Gray text indicates stretching muscles
- - - - indicates deep muscles

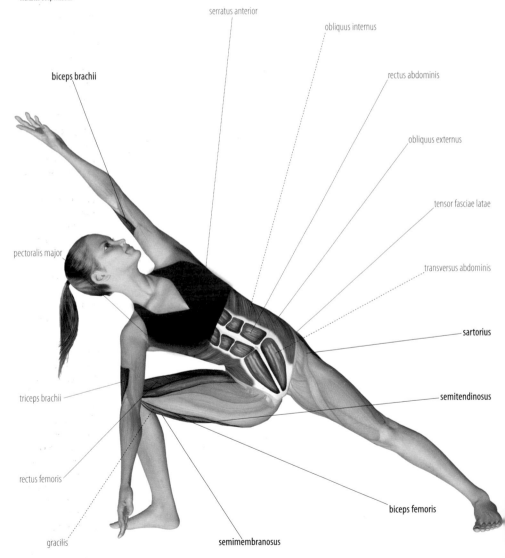

serratus anterior

obliquus internus

rectus abdominis

biceps brachii

obliquus externus

tensor fasciae latae

pectoralis major

transversus abdominis

sartorius

triceps brachii

semitendinosus

rectus femoris

biceps femoris

gracilis

semimembranosus

HOW TO DO IT

1 Stand in Virabhadrasana II (see pages 50–51), with your right leg bent, your left leg extended, and your arms raised to the sides, parallel to the floor.

2 Anchor your left heel to the floor. Your right knee should be bent over your right ankle, so that your shin is perpendicular to the floor. Aim the inside of your knee toward the outside of your foot. Bring your right thigh parallel to the floor.

3 Firm your shoulder blades against your back ribs. Extend your left arm straight up, and then turn your left palm to face toward your head. Inhale, and reach your left arm over the back of your left ear, palm facing the floor, stretching from your left heel through your left fingertips to lengthen the entire left side of your body. Make sure your elbow remains straight.

4 Turn your head to gaze at your left arm. Release your right shoulder away from your ear, creating as much length along the right side of your torso as you do along the left.

5 Continue to ground your left heel into the floor, exhale, and lay the right side of your torso down onto the top of your right thigh. Press your right fingertips or palm on the floor just outside of your right foot. Push your right knee back against your inner arm, while tucking your tailbone toward your pubis and pressing your hips forward.

6 Hold for 30 seconds to 1 minute.

7 Inhale, and begin to rise. Push both heels strongly into the floor, and reach your left arm toward the ceiling to lighten the upward movement. Reverse your feet, and repeat on the other side.

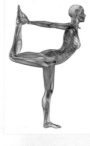

PRIMARY TARGETS
• semitendinosus
• semimembranosus
• obliquus internus
• transversus abdominis
• biceps femoris
• sartorius
• obliquus externus
• piriformis
• gracilis
• tensor fasciae latae

BENEFITS
• Strengthens legs, knees, and ankles
• Stretches legs, knees, ankles, groins, spine, waist, chest and lungs, and shoulders
• Stimulates abdominal organs
• Increases stamina

CAUTIONS
• Headache
• Insomnia
• High or low blood pressure

PERFECT YOUR FORM
• If you feel unsteady, brace your back heel against a wall.
• If you have trouble reaching the floor, place your right hand on a block, or bend your elbow and place your forearm on your right thigh, hand facing up, and your shoulder still away from your ear.

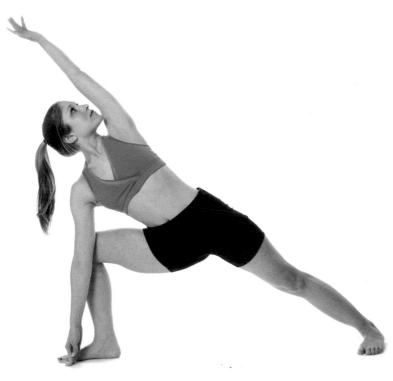

ANJANEYASANA

(Low Lunge; Crescent Moon Pose)

ANJANEYASANA, OR LOW LUNGE, is a foundation pose that will warm you up for more challenging asanas. Low Lunge, also known as the Crescent Moon Pose, is also a great stretch for tight quads, hamstrings, and hips and improves the strength and flexibility in your hips, legs, shoulders, arms, abdomen, back, and knees.

ANNOTATION KEY
Black text indicates strengthening muscles
Gray text indicates stretching muscles
- - - - indicates deep muscles

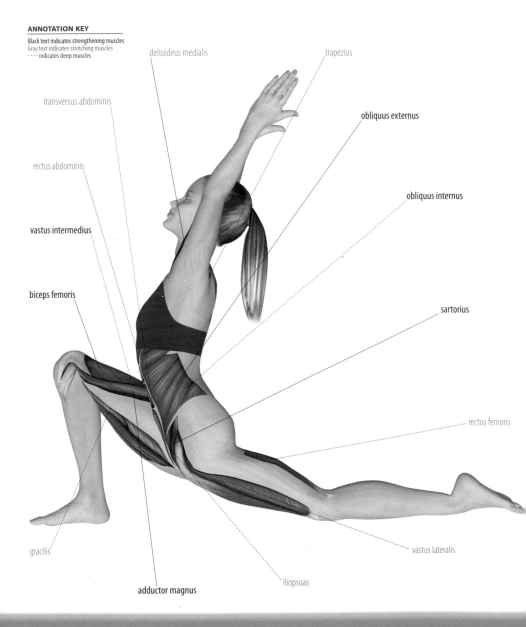

deltoideus medialis

trapezius

transversus abdominis

obliquus externus

rectus abdominis

obliquus internus

vastus intermedius

biceps femoris

sartorius

rectus femoris

gracilis

vastus lateralis

iliopsoas

adductor magnus

HOW TO DO IT

1 Stand in Adho Mukha Svanasana (see page 22). Exhale, and step your right foot forward between your hands, aligning your right knee over your heel.

2 Lower your left knee to the floor, and, keeping your right knee fixed in place, slide your left leg back until you feel a comfortable stretch in the front of your left thigh and groin. Rest the top of your left foot on the floor.

3 Inhale, and lift your torso to an upright position. At the same time, sweep your arms out to the sides and up toward the ceiling. Draw your tailbone down toward the floor, and lift your pubis toward your navel.

4 Tilt your head, and gaze upward while reaching your little fingers toward the ceiling. Hold for 1 minute.

5 Exhale, and fold your torso back down to your right thigh. Place your hands on the floor, and flip your toes so that the bottoms press against the floor. Exhale, and lift your left knee off the floor and step back to Adho Mukha Svanasana. Repeat on the other side.

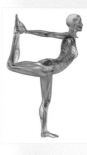

PRIMARY TARGETS
• rectus femoris
• obliquus internus
• obliquus externus
• biceps femoris
• deltoideus medialis
• trapezius
• sartorius
• adductor magnus
• iliopsoas

BENEFITS
• Relieves sciatica
• Tones hip abductors
• Strengthens arms and shoulders
• Stretches knee muscles, tendons, and ligaments

CAUTIONS
• Heart problems

PERFECT YOUR FORM
• Avoid dropping your knee to the inside or outside— it should remain forward, directly in front of you.
• If your lowered knee feels uncomfortable, place a folded towel underneath it.

VIRABHADRASANA I

BEGINNER

(Warrior I Pose)

THE GROUP OF ASANAS known as the Warrior Poses takes its name from the mythical Virabhadra, a fierce warrior who is said to have been an incarnation of the Hindu god Shiva. These beautiful moves display the practitioner's grace and strength. Warrior I is especially effective at increasing the flexibility of your hip flexors, the muscles at the front of your hips that pull your leg upward.

ANNOTATION KEY
Black text indicates strengthening muscles
Gray text indicates stretching muscles
- - - - indicates deep muscles

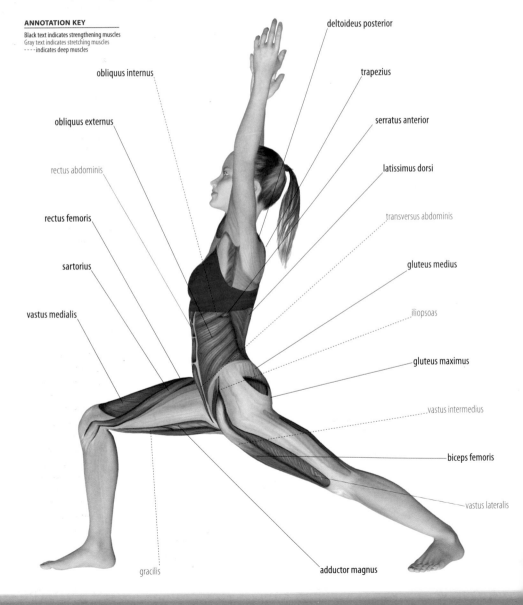

deltoideus posterior

obliquus internus

trapezius

obliquus externus

serratus anterior

rectus abdominis

latissimus dorsi

rectus femoris

transversus abdominis

sartorius

gluteus medius

vastus medialis

iliopsoas

gluteus maximus

vastus intermedius

biceps femoris

vastus lateralis

gracilis

adductor magnus

HOW TO DO IT

1 Stand in Tadasana (see pages 30–31). Exhale, and step your left foot back 3½ to 4 feet apart. Align your left heel behind your right heel, and then turn your left foot out 45 degrees, keeping you right foot facing straight forward. Rotate your hips so both hip bones are squared forward and are parallel to the front of your mat.

2 Inhale, and raise your arms toward the ceiling while keeping them parallel to each other and shoulder-width apart. Firm your shoulder blades against your back, and draw them down toward your tailbone.

3 Exhale, contract your abdominals, and tuck your tailbone under. With your left heel firmly grounded, exhale, and then slowly bend your right knee, stacking it over your heel. Your right shin should be perpendicular to the floor and your right thigh parallel to the floor.

4 Keep your head in a neutral position, gazing forward, or tilt it back and look up at your thumbs. Hold for 30 seconds to 1 minute.

5 To come up, inhale, press your back heel firmly into the floor and reach up with your arms, straightening your right knee. Turn your feet forward, exhale, and release your arms. Take a few breaths, turn your feet to the left, and repeat on the other side.

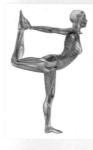

PRIMARY TARGETS

- rectus abdominis
- obliquus internus
- transversus abdominis
- biceps femoris
- sartorius
- obliquus externus

BENEFITS

- Strengthens arms, shoulders, thighs, ankles, and back
- Stretches hip flexors, abdominals, and ankles
- Expands chest, lungs, and shoulders
- Develops stamina
- Improves sense of balance

CAUTIONS

- Heart problems
- High blood pressure
- Shoulder injury

PERFECT YOUR FORM

- Avoid shifting your weight too far forward so that your front knee is aligned over your toes.
- Don't allow your hips to shift to either side.
- If you are a beginner, to maintain balance, decrease the distance between your feet by several inches, still keeping your right knee over your heel.

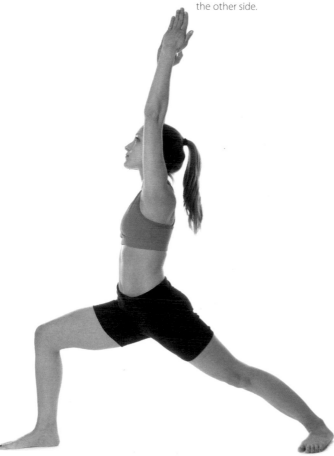

VIRABHADRASANA II

(Warrior II Pose)

ANOTHER GRACEFUL AND POWERFUL ASANA, Warrior II strengthens your legs and arms, opens your chest and shoulders, and tones your abdomen. To get the most from this pose, try to embody the might of a great warrior each time you perform it.

ANNOTATION KEY
Black text indicates strengthening muscles
Gray text indicates stretching muscles
----indicates deep muscles

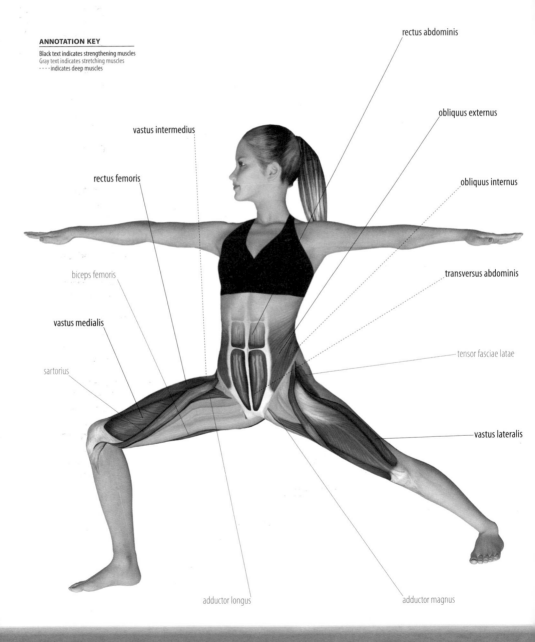

rectus abdominis

obliquus externus

vastus intermedius

obliquus internus

rectus femoris

transversus abdominis

biceps femoris

vastus medialis

tensor fasciae latae

sartorius

vastus lateralis

adductor longus

adductor magnus

HOW TO DO IT

1 Stand in Tadasana (see pages 30–31). Exhale, and step sideways so that your feet are 3½ to 4 feet apart.

2 Raise your arms parallel to the floor and reach them out to the sides with your shoulder blades wide and your palms facing downward.

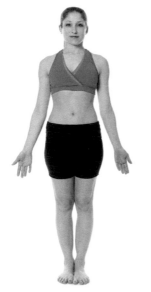

3 Turn your left foot in slightly to the right and your right foot out to the right 90 degrees. Align your right heel with your left heel. Firm your thighs and turn your right thigh outward so that the center of your right kneecap is in line with the center of your right ankle.

4 Exhale, and bend your right knee, so that your shin is perpendicular to the floor. Bring your right thigh parallel to the floor, anchoring your right knee by contracting the muscles of your left leg and pressing the outside of your left heel firmly to the floor. Keep the sides of your torso equally long and your shoulders aligned directly over your pelvis. Press your tailbone slightly toward your pubis.

5 Turn your head to the right and look out over your fingers.

6 Hold for 30 seconds to 1 minute. Inhale, and return to Tadasana. Reverse your feet and repeat on the other side.

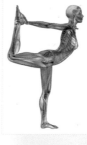

PRIMARY TARGETS
- gluteus maximus
- gluteus medius
- obliquus externus
- biceps femoris
- sartorius
- adductor longus
- adductor magnus
- sartorius

BENEFITS
- Strengthens legs and ankles
- Stretches legs, ankles, groins, chest, and shoulders
- Stimulates digestion
- Increases stamina
- Relieves backache
- Relieves carpal tunnel syndrome
- Relieves sciatica

CAUTIONS
- Diarrhea
- High blood pressure
- Neck issues

PERFECT YOUR FORM
- Focus on turning the knee of your bent leg outward, opening your hips and groins.
- Avoid allowing your knee to drift over to either side.
- Avoid leaning your torso over your bent leg.

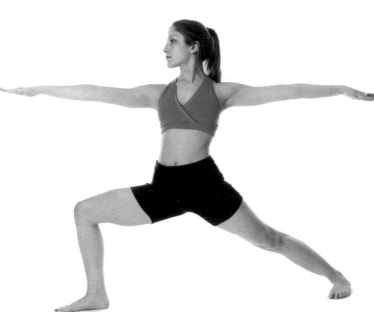

VIRABHADRASANA III

INTERMEDIATE

(Warrior III Pose)

WHEN PROPERLY PERFORMED, Warrior III makes the yoga practitioner look as if she is about to take flight. This powerful pose tones your abdominals and increases your sense of balance and will leave you feeling strong and centered.

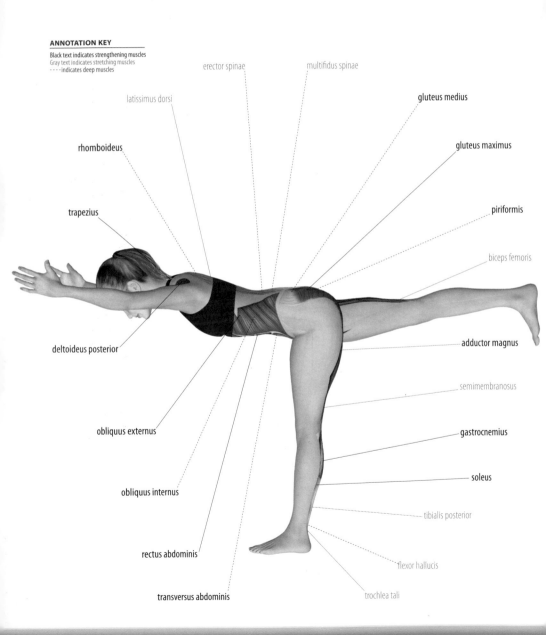

ANNOTATION KEY

Black text indicates strengthening muscles
Gray text indicates stretching muscles
- - - - indicates deep muscles

erector spinae

multifidus spinae

latissimus dorsi

gluteus medius

rhomboideus

gluteus maximus

trapezius

piriformis

biceps femoris

deltoideus posterior

adductor magnus

semimembranosus

obliquus externus

gastrocnemius

obliquus internus

soleus

tibialis posterior

rectus abdominis

flexor hallucis

transversus abdominis

trochlea tali

HOW TO DO IT

1 Stand in Tadasana (see pages 30–31). Exhale, and step your right foot about 1 foot forward, shifting all of your weight onto your right leg.

2 Inhale, and raise your arms over your head, interlacing your fingers and pointing your index fingers upward.

3 Exhale, and lift your left leg up behind you, hinging at your hips to lower your arms and torso down toward the floor.

4 Gaze down at a point on the floor for balance. Elongate your body from your left toes through the crown of your head to your fingers, making one straight line.

5 Hold for 30 seconds to 1 minute.

6 Inhale, and raise your arms upward as you lower your left leg back to the floor. Bring both feet together into Tadasana.

7 Repeat on the other side.

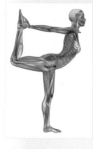

PRIMARY TARGETS
• rectus abdominis
• obliquus internus
• transversus abdominis
• biceps femoris
• erector spinae
• gluteus maximus
• deltoideus posterior

BENEFITS
• Strengthens ankles, legs, shoulders, and back muscles
• Tones abdominals
• Improves sense of balance
• Improves posture

CAUTIONS
• High blood pressure

PERFECT YOUR FORM
• Position your arms, torso, and raised leg relatively parallel to the floor.
• Avoid tilting your pelvis so that your hips are not aligned.
• Avoid compressing the back of your neck.

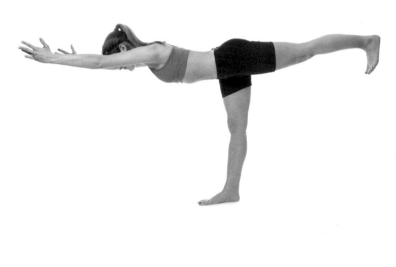

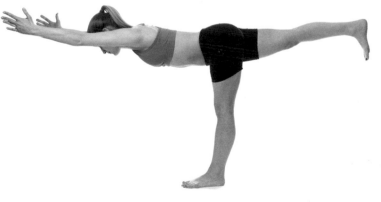

HIGH LUNGE

INTERMEDIATE

HIGH LUNGE IS AN EFFECTIVE leg and arm strengthener that will also stretch your groins. Although some schools of yoga call it Ashva Sanchalanasana, which roughly translates from the Sanskrit as "Horse Rider's Pose" or "Equestrian Pose," there is no generally agreed-upon Sanskrit name for this pose.

ANNOTATION KEY
Black text indicates strengthening muscles
Gray text indicates stretching muscles
- - - -indicates deep muscles

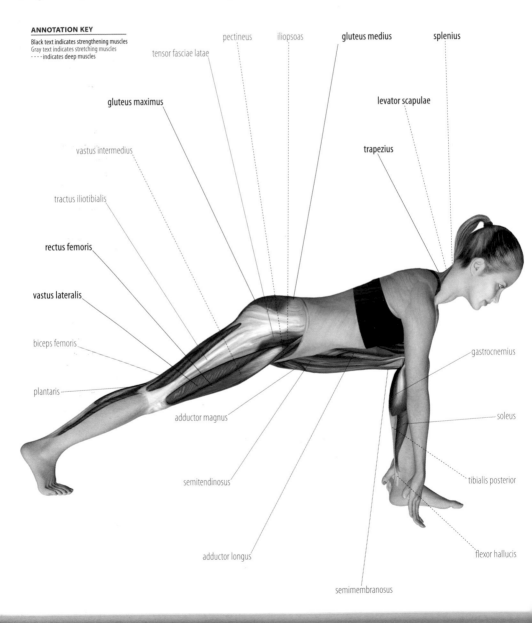

pectineus

iliopsoas

gluteus medius

splenius

tensor fasciae latae

levator scapulae

gluteus maximus

trapezius

vastus intermedius

tractus iliotibialis

rectus femoris

vastus lateralis

biceps femoris

gastrocnemius

plantaris

soleus

adductor magnus

tibialis posterior

semitendinosus

flexor hallucis

adductor longus

semimembranosus

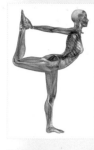

HOW TO DO IT

1 Stand in Tadasana (see pages 30–31), and inhale deeply. Exhale, and then carefully step back with your left leg, keeping it in line with your hips as you step back. The ball of your left foot should be in contact with the floor as you do the motion.

2 Slowly slide your left foot farther back, while bending your right knee, stacking it directly above your ankle.

3 Position your palms or fingertips on the floor on either side of your right leg, and slowly press your palms or fingertips against the floor to enhance the placement of your upper body and your head.

4 Lift your head, and gaze straight forward, leaning your upper body forward and carefully rolling your shoulders down and backward.

5 Press the ball of your left foot gradually into the floor, contract your thigh muscles, and press up to maintain your left leg in a straight position.

6 Hold for 5 to 6 seconds, and then slowly return to Tadasana. Repeat on the other side.

PRIMARY TARGETS
• biceps femoris
• adductor longus
• adductor magnus
• gastrocnemius
• tibialis posterior
• iliopsoas
• biceps femoris
• rectus femoris

BENEFITS
• Strengthens legs and arms
• Stretches groins
• Relieves constipation

CAUTIONS
• Arm injury
• Shoulder injury
• Hip injury
• High or low blood pressure
• Severe headache

PERFECT YOUR FORM
• Maintain proper position of your shoulders and your whole upper body to lengthen your spine.
• Avoid dropping your back-extended knee to the floor.

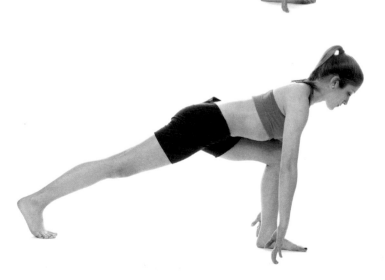

UTTHITA HASTA PADANGUSTHASANA

INTERMEDIATE

(Extended Hand-to-Big-Toe Pose)

UTTHITA HASTA PADANGUSTANA, or Extended Hand-to-Big-Toe Pose, requires the solid grounding of your standing foot to keep you steady. As well as helping you to improve your balance, this asana stretches your hamstrings and keeps your legs limber.

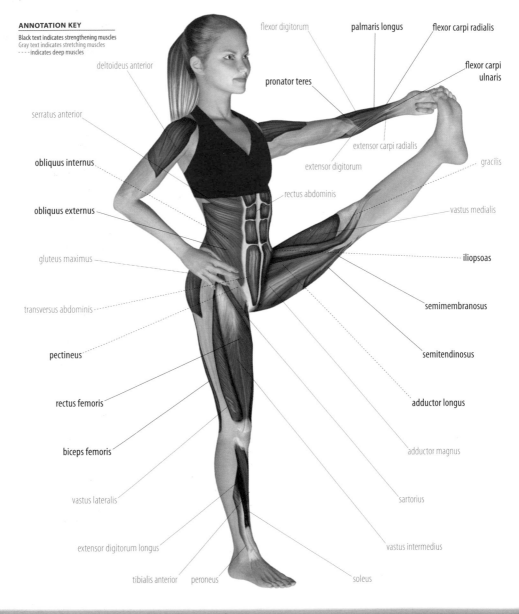

ANNOTATION KEY
Black text indicates strengthening muscles
Gray text indicates stretching muscles
----indicates deep muscles

flexor digitorum

palmaris longus

flexor carpi radialis

deltoideus anterior

pronator teres

flexor carpi ulnaris

serratus anterior

extensor carpi radialis

obliquus internus

extensor digitorum

gracilis

rectus abdominis

obliquus externus

vastus medialis

gluteus maximus

iliopsoas

transversus abdominis

semimembranosus

pectineus

semitendinosus

rectus femoris

adductor longus

biceps femoris

adductor magnus

vastus lateralis

sartorius

extensor digitorum longus

vastus intermedius

tibialis anterior   peroneus

soleus

HOW TO DO IT

1 Stand in Tadasana (see pages 30–31). Shift your weight onto your right foot. Firmly ground your right foot, pressing all corners of your foot and toes into the floor.

2 Square your hips facing forward, and raise your left leg toward your chest by bending your left knee. Grasp your left big toe with two fingers of your left hand curled around it. Rest your right hand on your right hip.

3 Exhale, and extend your left leg, straightening it while pulling your foot inward as your extended leg moves to come in line with your torso.

4 Gaze at a single spot on the floor about a body's length in front of you. Flex your foot so that your toes curl back toward you. Hold for about 30 seconds.

5 Exhale, and lower your foot to the floor. Repeat on the other side.

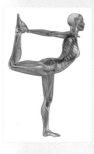

PRIMARY TARGETS
- rectus femoris
- vastus lateralis
- vastus medialis
- pronator teres
- flexor carpi radialis
- palmaris longus
- biceps femoris
- semitendinosus
- semimembranosus
- quadratus lumborum
- piriformis
- gemellus superior
- gemellus inferior
- tibialis anterior
- gracilis
- gluteus maximus

BENEFITS
- Strengthens legs and ankles
- Stretches backs of the legs
- Improves sense of balance

CAUTIONS
- Ankle injury
- Lower-back injury

PERFECT YOUR FORM
- Keep your hips squared, facing forward, even when you raise your leg.
- Extend your torso, keeping as much space between your sternum and pubic bone as possible.

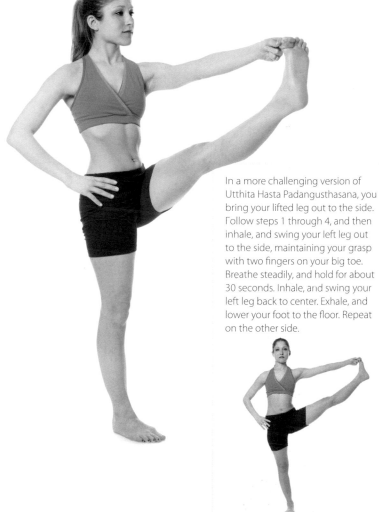

In a more challenging version of Utthita Hasta Padangusthasana, you bring your lifted leg out to the side. Follow steps 1 through 4, and then inhale, and swing your left leg out to the side, maintaining your grasp with two fingers on your big toe. Breathe steadily, and hold for about 30 seconds. Inhale, and swing your left leg back to center. Exhale, and lower your foot to the floor. Repeat on the other side.

ARDHA CHANDRASANA

INTERMEDIATE

(Half Moon Pose)

ARDHA CHANDRASANA, or Half Moon Pose, challenges you to balance all your weight between your five fingers and one foot. It is essential to really root down through your standing leg while allowing your torso, top arm, and top leg to float above. If you are just learning this asana, press your back foot into a wall while finding your center of balance.

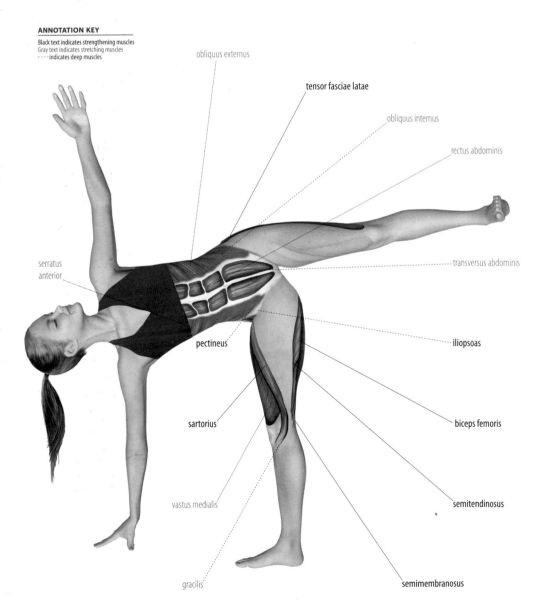

ANNOTATION KEY
Black text indicates strengthening muscles
Gray text indicates stretching muscles
----indicates deep muscles

obliquus externus

tensor fasciae latae

obliquus internus

rectus abdominis

serratus anterior

transversus abdominis

pectineus

iliopsoas

sartorius

biceps femoris

vastus medialis

semitendinosus

gracilis

semimembranosus

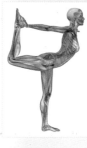

HOW TO DO IT

1 Stand in Trikonasana (see pages 42–43) to the right side, and rest your left hand on your left hip.

2 Inhale, and with your right knee still bent, slide your left foot forward about 6 to 12 inches. At the same time, reach your right hand forward, beyond the little-toe side of your right foot, at least 12 inches.

3 Exhale, press your right hand and right heel firmly into the floor, and straighten your right leg, simultaneously lifting your left leg parallel to the floor.

4 Rotate your upper torso to the left, while moving your left hip slightly forward. Most of your weight should rest on your standing leg. Press your right hand lightly against the floor, using it to maintain your balance.

5 Hold for 30 seconds to 1 minute. Exhale, lower your raised leg to the floor, and return to Trikonasana. Repeat on the other side, starting with your left leg.

PRIMARY TARGETS
- latissimus dorsi
- obliquus internus
- obliquus externus
- serratus anterior
- transversus abdominis
- rectus abdominis
- vastus medialis
- biceps femoris

BENEFITS
- Strengthens spine, abdominals, ankles, thighs, and buttocks
- Stretches groins, hamstrings, calves, shoulders, chest, and spine
- Improves sense of balance
- Relieves stress
- Stimulates digestion

CAUTIONS
- Headache
- Diarrhea
- Low blood pressure

PERFECT YOUR FORM
- Don't lock your standing knee.
- Avoid turning the kneecap of your standing leg inward—your kneecap should be aligned straight forward.

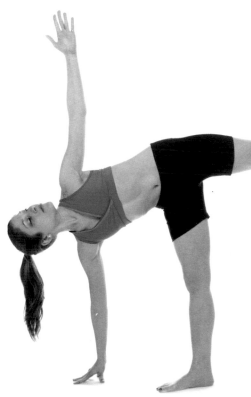

PARIVRTTA TRIKONASANA

INTERMEDIATE

(Revolved Triangle Pose)

A STANDING BALANCE, forward bend, and twist, Parivrtta Trikonasana, or Revolved Triangle Pose, adds rotation to the basic Trikonasana. It's a challenging standing pose that stretches the muscles of your outer hip and lengthens your hamstrings, while toning your legs, back, and obliques. Balancing your pelvis is essential to proper alignment.

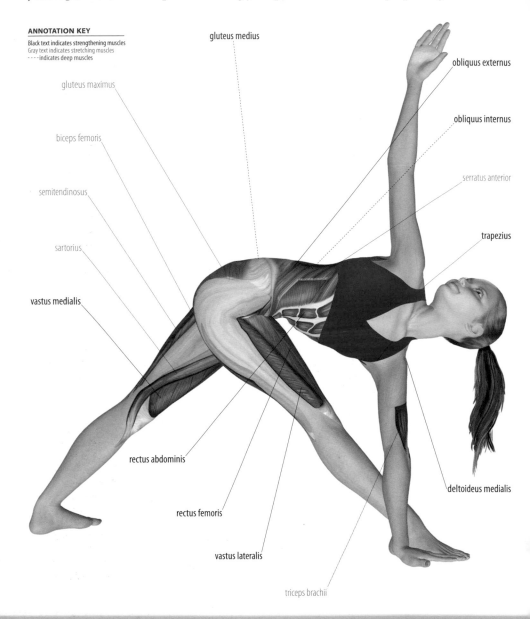

ANNOTATION KEY

Black text indicates strengthening muscles
Gray text indicates stretching muscles
----indicates deep muscles

gluteus medius

obliquus externus

obliquus internus

serratus anterior

trapezius

gluteus maximus

biceps femoris

semitendinosus

sartorius

vastus medialis

rectus abdominis

rectus femoris

vastus lateralis

deltoideus medialis

triceps brachii

HOW TO DO IT

1 Stand in Tadasana (see pages 30–31). Exhale, and step or lightly jump your feet 3½ to 4 feet apart.

2 Raise your arms parallel to the floor and reach them out to the sides, with your shoulder blades wide, palms down. Turn your left foot in 45 to 60 degrees to the right and your right foot out 90 degrees to the right. Align your heels with each other, contract your thigh muscles, and turn your right thigh outward, so that the center of your right kneecap is in line with the center of your right ankle.

3 Exhale, and turn your torso to the right, squaring your hip points with the front edge of your mat. As you bring your left hip around to the right, firmly ground your left heel. Inhale.

4 Exhale, and turn your torso farther to the right, leaning forward over your front leg. Reach your left hand down, either to the floor or on either side of your right foot. Allow your left hip to drop slightly toward the floor.

5 Turn your head to gaze upward at your top thumb. Widen the space between your shoulder blades, pressing your arms away from your torso. Shift most of your weight to your back heel and front hand.

6 Hold for 30 seconds to 1 minute. Exhale, release the twist, and bring your torso upright with an inhalation. Repeat for the same length of time with the legs reversed, twisting to the left.

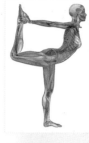

PRIMARY TARGETS
- rectus femoris
- biceps femoris
- gluteus maximus
- gluteus medius
- obliquus internus
- obliquus externus
- latissimus dorsi
- erector spinae

BENEFITS
- Strengthens legs
- Stretches groins, hamstrings, and hips
- Opens chest and shoulders

CAUTIONS
- Low blood pressure
- Migraine
- Diarrhea
- Insomnia

PERFECT YOUR FORM
- Keep your hips level and parallel to the floor.
- If your are a beginner, rather than gaze upward, keep your head in a neutral position, looking straight forward, or turn your head to look at the floor.
- If you feel your hip slip out to the side and lift up toward your shoulder, press your outer right thigh actively to the left and release your right hip away from your right shoulder.

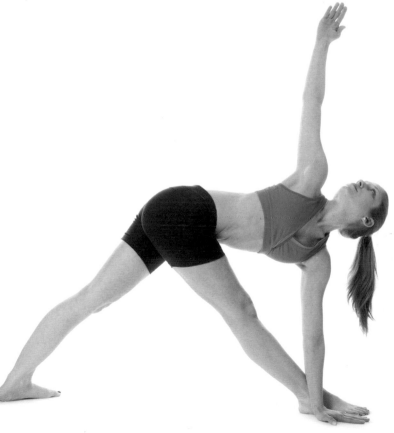

URDHVA PRASARITA EKA PADASANA

ADVANCED

(Standing Splits; One Foot Extended Upwards Pose)

URDHVA PRASARITA EKA PADASANA, or Standing Splits, tones your entire body and efficiently stretches you from neck to ankle. It's also particularly effective at firming and lifting your glutes. To get the most from this asana, try to move your feet away from each other rather than just lifting your back foot.

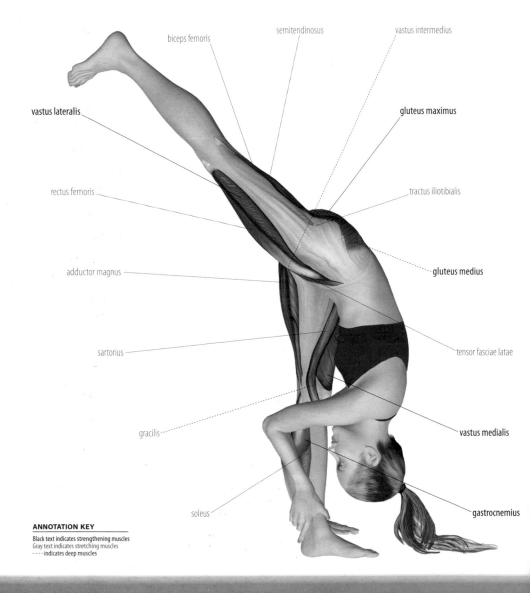

biceps femoris

semitendinosus

vastus intermedius

vastus lateralis

gluteus maximus

rectus femoris

tractus iliotibialis

adductor magnus

gluteus medius

sartorius

tensor fasciae latae

gracilis

vastus medialis

soleus

gastrocnemius

ANNOTATION KEY

Black text indicates strengthening muscles
Gray text indicates stretching muscles
- - - - indicates deep muscles

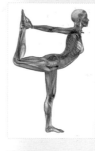

HOW TO DO IT

1 Stand in Tadasana (see pages 30–31), and shift your weight onto your left foot.

2 Bend forward with your back flat, simultaneously raising your right leg behind you. Square your shoulders and your hips forward. Reach your fingertips to the floor.

3 Exhale, and contract your leg muscles as you fold your torso onto your left thigh. Lift your right heel toward the ceiling, extending both legs in opposite directions as far as you are able.

4 Relax your shoulders toward the floor. In this position, your left knee is pointed forward and your right knee is pointed straight behind you. If possible, grasp the back of your left ankle with your right hand. Maintain balance with your left palm on the floor.

5 Hold for 30 seconds to 1 minute. Repeat on the other side.

Challenge ourself with this deeper version of the Standing Split: Follow steps 1 through 4, and then extend the split farther by turning your hip slightly outward, so that your right knee points to the right. Keep your left leg straight and firmly grounded. Reach your toes toward the ceiling by continuously kicking gently upward with your back leg.

PRIMARY TARGETS
• biceps femoris
• semitendinosus
• sartorius
• rectus femoris
• tensor fasciae latae
• gluteus maximus
• gastrocnemius

BENEFITS
• Stretches groins, thighs, and calves
• Strengthens thighs, knees, and ankles
• Improves balance

CAUTIONS
• Lower-back injury
• Ankle injury
• Knee injury

PERFECT YOUR FORM
• Lower your torso, and lift your back leg simultaneously.
• Tuck your chin, and elongate the back of your neck.
• Avoid rotating your standing knee inward.
• Avoid rounding your spine.
• Don't bend forward from your waist.

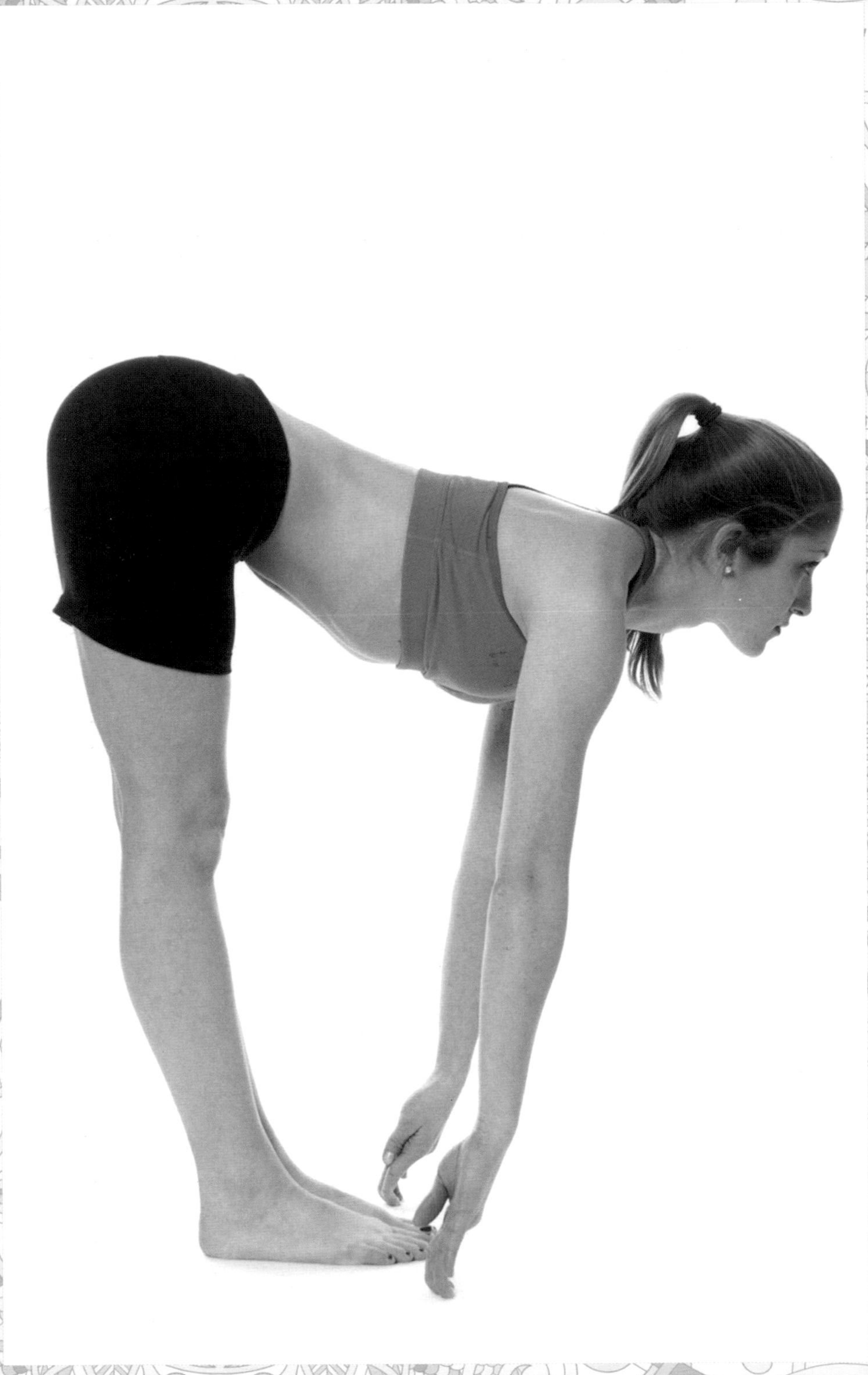

FORWARD BENDS

Forward bends may be as straightforward as yoga poses come, but they are certainly not lacking in variety. Both seated and standing, forward bends include poses with the legs together and separated—either out to the side or in opposition to each other.

All of the poses in this section will challenge your body's sense of alignment. Forward bends will stretch your hamstrings and the entire back of your body, releasing your spine. It is important to bend at your hips rather than your waist, because bending at your waist will shorten your movement and strain your back. To do this, flatten your back and fold—don't curl—into the pose.

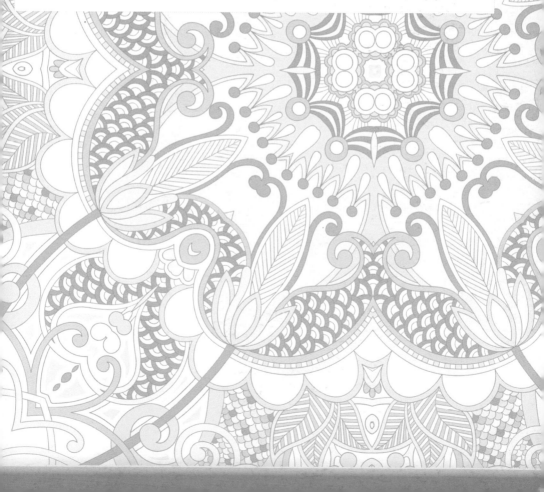

UTTANASANA TO ARDHA UTTANASANA

BEGINNER *(Standing Forward Bend to Standing Half Forward Bend)*

STAYING LIMBER is an essential component of yoga practice. Both Uttanasana and Ardha Uttanasana—Standing Forward Bend and Standing Half Forward Bend—work your quadriceps to stretch your hamstrings, calf muscles, and lower back. Also working your abdominals, these revitalizing asanas are part of the Sun Salutations.

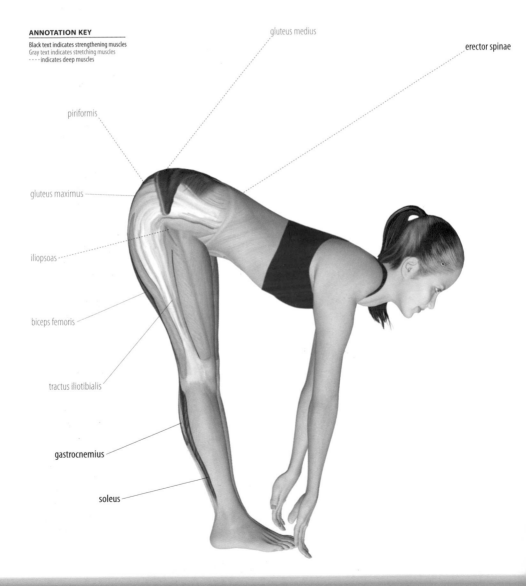

ANNOTATION KEY
Black text indicates strengthening muscles
Gray text indicates stretching muscles
---- indicates deep muscles

gluteus medius

erector spinae

piriformis

gluteus maximus

iliopsoas

biceps femoris

tractus iliotibialis

gastrocnemius

soleus

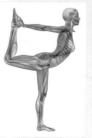

HOW TO DO IT

1 Stand in Tadasana (see pages 30–31), and then raise your arms toward the ceiling in Utkatasana (see page 34–35).

2 Exhale, and bend forward from your hips, sweeping your arms to the sides with your palms facing the floor. While you lower your torso, keep your back flat, and tuck your abdominals in toward your spine. Lengthen your spine as much as possible.

3 Fold your torso onto the front of your legs, aiming your forehead toward your shins. Grasp the backs of your ankles, and contract your thigh muscles to straighten your knees.

4 With each exhalation, draw your sit bones upward, and elongate your spine to the floor even more to create a deeper stretch.

5 Hold for 30 seconds to 1 minute.

6 From Uttanasana, move into Ardha Uttanasana by placing your hands beside your feet. Inhale, and lift your head and upper torso away from your legs, keeping your back flat. Straighten your elbows and use your fingertips to guide your lift.

7 Lift your chest forward, elongating your spine into a slight arch. Lengthen the back of your neck as you gaze forward.

8 Hold for 10 to 30 seconds. Lower yourself back to Uttanasana, or inhale, and lift your torso all the way back up to stand in Tadasana.

PRIMARY TARGETS
- biceps femoris
- tractus iliotibialis
- gluteus maximus
- gluteus medius
- erector spinae

BENEFITS
- Stretches spine, hamstrings, calves, and hips
- Strengthens spine and thighs
- Improves posture
- Relieves stress

CAUTIONS
- Back injury
- Neck injury
- Osteoporosis

PERFECT YOUR FORM
- If you have tight hamstrings, bend your knees as you fold your torso forward. Work on pressing your knees straight once you are in the forward bend. You may also bend your knees on your way up to Ardha Uttanasana to help create a slight arch In your back.
- Avoid rolling your spine into or out of the pose.
- Avoid compressing the back of your neck as you look forward.

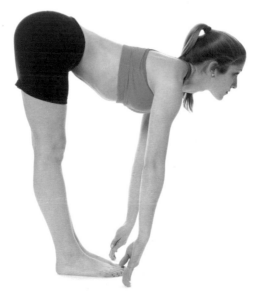

BADDHA KONASANA

BEGINNER *(Bound Angle Pose; Butterfly Pose; Cobbler's Pose)*

BADDHA KONASANA, or Bound Angle Pose, opens the hips and groins. Your goal will be to get your knees on the floor, but don't rush to achieve it. Work gradually to improve the flexibility of your hips and groin until this pose becomes second nature. If you are a more advanced practitioner, you can add a deeper forward bend by folding your torso flat over your legs so that your head rests in front of your feet.

ANNOTATION KEY
Black text indicates strengthening muscles
Gray text indicates stretching muscles
- - - - indicates deep muscles

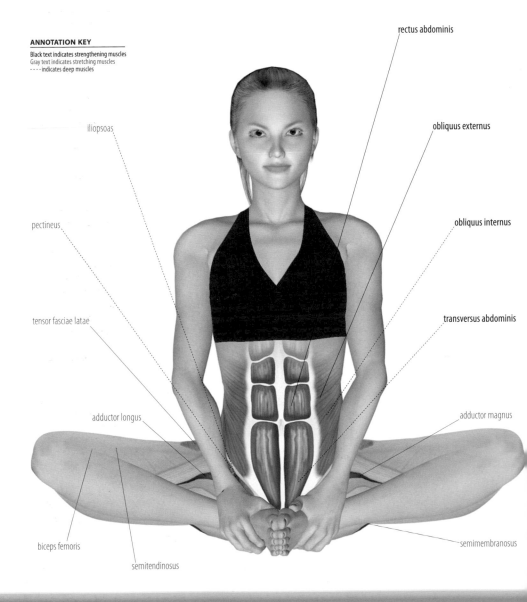

rectus abdominis

obliquus externus

obliquus internus

transversus abdominis

iliopsoas

pectineus

tensor fasciae latae

adductor longus

adductor magnus

biceps femoris

semitendinosus

semimembranosus

HOW TO DO IT

1 Sit up tall in Dandasana (see page 19), with your legs extended in front of you and with your shoulders relaxed.

2 Bring your knees toward your chest with your feet flat on the floor.

3 Exhale, and open your hips, drawing your thighs to the floor. Use your hands to press your feet together, and keep the outsides of your feet on the floor.

4 Draw your torso upward, and focus on keeping your spine in a neutral position. Your weight should be balanced evenly on your sit bones. Allow your hips to open farther and your thighs to drop to the floor.

5 Hold for 1 to 5 minutes.

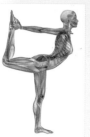

PRIMARY TARGETS
- iliopsoas
- tensor fasciae latae
- adductor magnus
- adductor longus

BENEFITS
- Stretches inner thighs, groins, and knees
- Provides relief from menstrual discomfort

CAUTIONS
- Knee injury
- Groin injury

PERFECT YOUR FORM
- Lift upward from your spine, and keep your chest and shoulders pressed open, creating a straight line from your sit bones to your shoulders.
- If your groins and inner thighs are tight, place a folded blanket beneath your buttocks.
- To deepen the stretch, bend forward, leading with your chest.
- Avoid pushing your knees down with your hands.
- Avoid rounding the back of your neck as you look forward.

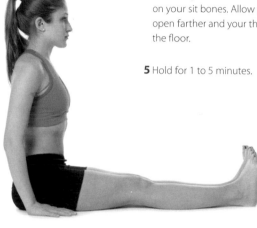

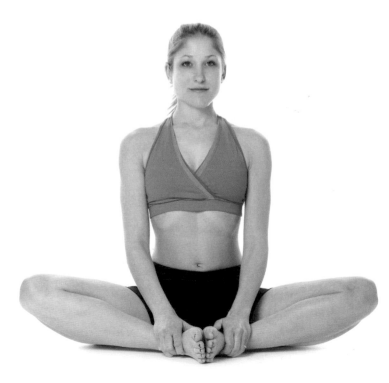

JANU SIRSASANA

BEGINNER

*(Head-to-Knee Pose; Head-to-Knee Forward Bend;
Head of the Knee Pose; Head-on-Knee Pose)*

A FORWARD BEND for all levels of students, Janu Sirsasana goes by many names—Head-to-Knee Pose, Head-to-Knee Forward Bend, Head of the Knee Pose, or Head-on-Knee Pose. As well as a forward bend, it also works as a spinal twist and is one of the primary asanas of the Ashtanga school of yoga. To make the move easier as you work on your flexibility, you can hook a strap around your extended foot and hold an end in each hand as you bend forward. Placing a folded blanket under your buttocks will also decrease the amount of forward bend you need in your hips.

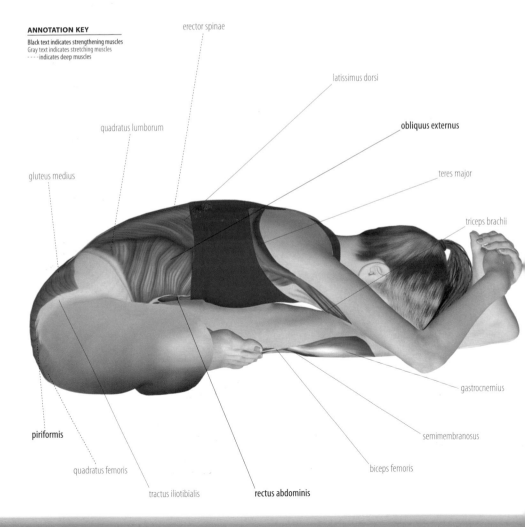

ANNOTATION KEY

Black text indicates strengthening muscles
Gray text indicates stretching muscles
- - - - indicates deep muscles

erector spinae

latissimus dorsi

obliquus externus

quadratus lumborum

teres major

gluteus medius

triceps brachii

gastrocnemius

piriformis

semimembranosus

quadratus femoris

biceps femoris

tractus iliotibialis

rectus abdominis

HOW TO DO IT

1 Begin in Dandasana (see page 19). Bend your right knee, and draw your heel toward your groin, placing the sole of your foot on your left inner thigh. Lower your right knee to the floor. Your left leg should sit at a right angle to your right shin. Draw both sit bones to the floor.

2 Inhale, and lift up through your spine. Turn your torso slightly to your left as you exhale so that it aligns with your left leg. Flex your foot, and contract the muscles in your left thigh to push the back of your leg toward the floor.

3 With another exhalation, stretch your sternum forward as you fold your torso over your left leg. Grasp the inside of your left foot with your right hand. Use your left hand to guide your torso to the left.

4 Extend your left arm forward toward your left foot. You may grasp your foot with both hands or place your hands on the floor on either side of your foot with your elbows bent. If possible, place your forehead on your left shin. With each inhalation, lengthen your spine, and with each exhalation, deepen the stretch.

5 Hold for 1 to 3 minutes. Repeat with your right leg bent.

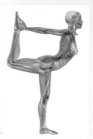

PRIMARY TARGETS
- biceps femoris
- gastrocnemius
- semimembranosus
- quadratus femoris
- tractus iliotibialis
- latissimus dorsi

BENEFITS
- Stretches hamstrings, groins, and spine
- Stimulates digestion
- Relieves headaches
- Alleviates high blood pressure

CAUTIONS
- Knee injury
- Lower-back injury
- Diarrhea

PERFECT YOUR FORM
- While bending forward, your abdominals should be the first parts of your body to touch your thigh. Your head should be the last.
- Don't allow the foot of your bent leg to shift beneath your straight leg.

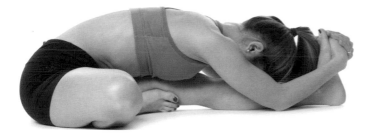

Paschimottanasana, or Seated Forward Bend, is similar to Janu Sirsasana. To get into this pose, sit in Dandasana, and then rock back and forth slightly to draw your sit bones as far away from your heels as possible. Flex your feet, and contract your thighs to press the backs of your legs against the floor. Inhale, and lift your arms straight up, lengthening your spine. Exhale, and stretch your sternum forward, bending from your hips. With your head forward, lower your abdominals to your thighs. Grasp the soles of your feet or your ankles with your hands. With each inhalation, lengthen your spine to deepen the stretch. If possible, bend your elbows to gently lengthen your torso forward, and place your forehead on your shins. Hold for 1 to 3 minutes.

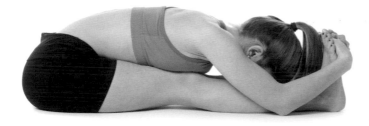

PRASARITA PADOTTANASANA

(Wide-Angle Standing Forward Bend;
Wide-Legged Forward Bend; Standing Straddle Forward Bend)

PRASARITA PADOTTANASANA stretches your entire body, with particular focus on your hamstrings and spine. Known also as Wide-Angle Standing Forward Bend, Wide-Legged Forward Bend, and Standing Straddle Forward Bend, this asana grounds your body while opening your hips and calming your mind.

ANNOTATION KEY
Black text indicates strengthening muscles
Gray text indicates stretching muscles
- - - - indicates deep muscles

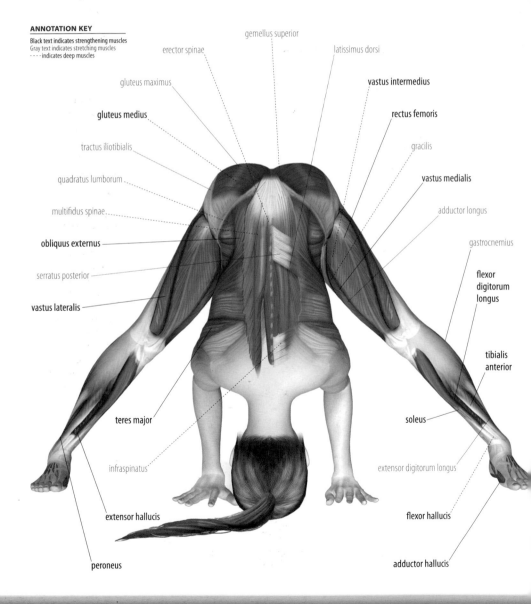

gemellus superior

erector spinae

latissimus dorsi

vastus intermedius

gluteus maximus

rectus femoris

gluteus medius

gracilis

tractus iliotibialis

vastus medialis

quadratus lumborum

adductor longus

multifidus spinae

gastrocnemius

obliquus externus

flexor digitorum longus

serratus posterior

vastus lateralis

tibialis anterior

teres major

soleus

infraspinatus

extensor digitorum longus

extensor hallucis

flexor hallucis

peroneus

adductor hallucis

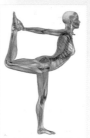

HOW TO DO IT

1 Stand in Tadasana (see pages 30–31). Take a large step—about 3 to 4 feet—to the side. Your feet should be parallel to each other. Lift up through your spine, and contract your thigh muscles.

2 Exhale, and bend forward from your hips, keeping your back flat. Draw your sternum forward as you lower your torso, gazing straight ahead. With your elbows straight, place your fingertips on the floor.

3 With another exhalation, place your hands on the floor in between your feet, and lower your torso into a full forward bend. Lengthen your spine by pulling your sit bones up toward the ceiling and drawing your head to the floor. If possible, bend your elbows and place your forehead on the floor.

4 Hold for 30 seconds to 1 minute. To release, straighten your elbows and raise your torso while keeping your back flat.

PRIMARY TARGETS
• gluteus maximus
• biceps femoris
• semitendinosus
• adductor longus
• adductor magnus
• tibialis anterior
• erector spinae

BENEFITS
• Stretches and strengthens hamstrings, groins, and spine

CAUTIONS
• Lower-back issues

PERFECT YOUR FORM
• Contract your leg muscles, and ground your feet throughout the pose.
• If you have trouble reaching your hands to the floor, widen your stance or place blocks on the floor for support.
• Don't bend forward from your waist.

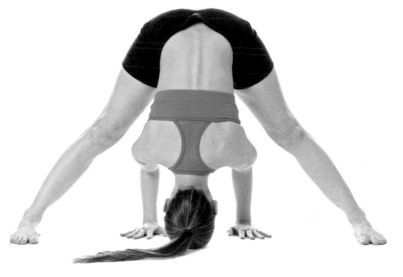

If you are not yet flexible enough to reach your head to the floor, try this easier version of Prasarita Padottanasana: Follow step 1, and then exhale, bending forward until your torso is nearly parallel to the ground. Place your hands on the ground in line with your shoulders, making sure that your lower back is straight. Hold for 30 seconds to 1 minute.

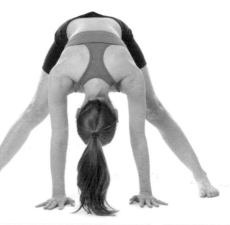

UPAVISTHA KONASANA

INTERMEDIATE *(Wide-Angle Seated Forward Bend; Seated Wide-Legged Straddle)*

UPAVISTHA KONASANA, known also as the Wide-Angle Seated Forward Bend or Seated Wide-Legged Straddle, is a challenging asana that stretches your hip adductor muscles and hamstrings. For those who are limber enough to relax into it, Upavistha Konasana is a restful posture in which you sit comfortably with your legs spread wide, your torso stretched out long between your legs, and your head resting on the floor with your neck and jaw muscles soft. While in this pose, remember to breathe deeply and fully, allowing yourself to fully relax your mind and body.

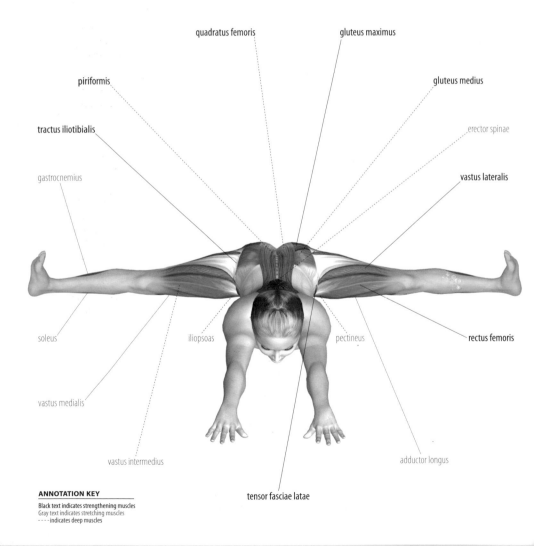

quadratus femoris

gluteus maximus

piriformis

gluteus medius

tractus iliotibialis

erector spinae

gastrocnemius

vastus lateralis

soleus

iliopsoas

pectineus

rectus femoris

vastus medialis

vastus intermedius

adductor longus

tensor fasciae latae

ANNOTATION KEY
Black text indicates strengthening muscles
Gray text indicates stretching muscles
----indicates deep muscles

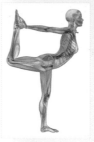

HOW TO DO IT

1 Sit in Dandasana (see page 19).

2 Separate your legs as wide as you can comfortably stretch. Turn your thighs slightly outward so that your knees point toward the ceiling. Flex your feet. Place your hands on the floor behind your buttocks to push them forward, separating your legs even farther.

3 Inhale, and lift up with your torso, placing your hands on the floor in front

of you. Contract your leg muscles, and press the backs of your thighs and both sit bones into the floor.

4 Exhale, and bend forward from your waist, keeping your back flat. Walk your hands in front of you to lower your torso slowly toward the floor. Gaze forward. Stretch as far as possible without rounding your back.

5 Hold for 1 to 2 minutes.

PRIMARY TARGETS
- erector spinae
- piriformis
- gluteus medius
- gracilis
- semitendinosus
- semimembranosus
- biceps femoris
- adductor longus
- adductor magnus

BENEFITS
- Stretches groins and hamstrings
- Strengthens spine

CAUTIONS
- Headache
- Diarrhea

PERFECT YOUR FORM
- If you have trouble bending forward from your hips, place a folded blanket beneath your buttocks.
- Avoid forcing your torso to the ground.

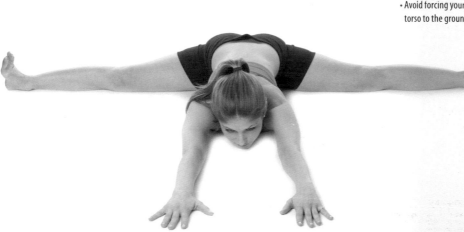

PARSVOTTANASANA

INTERMEDIATE

(Intense Side Stretch; Pyramid Pose)

PARSVOTTANASANA IS AN ASYMMETRICAL standing forward bend that offers a whole-body stretch, hence one of its other names—the Intense Side Stretch Pose. Also known as the Pyramid Pose, this asana offers the benefits of three major kinds of yoga movements: forward bending that stretches the hamstrings, glutes, and calf muscles; backward bending that releases your shoulder girdle and upper-back muscles and stretches your wrists and forearms; and balancing, which improves your coordination.

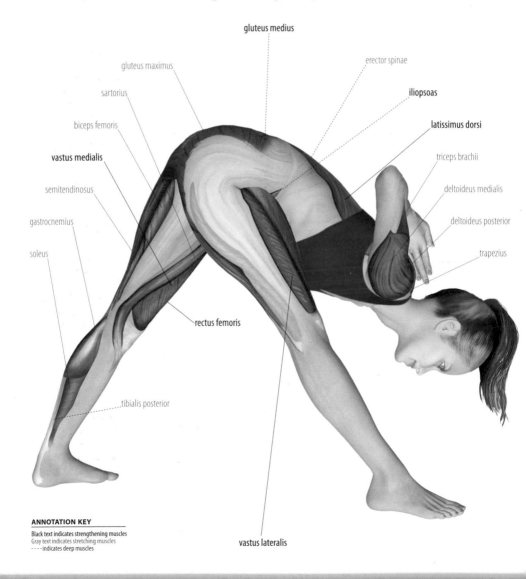

gluteus medius

erector spinae

gluteus maximus

iliopsoas

sartorius

latissimus dorsi

biceps femoris

triceps brachii

vastus medialis

deltoideus medialis

semitendinosus

deltoideus posterior

gastrocnemius

trapezius

soleus

rectus femoris

tibialis posterior

ANNOTATION KEY

Black text indicates strengthening muscles
Gray text indicates stretching muscles
- - - - indicates deep muscles

vastus lateralis

HOW TO DO IT

1 Stand in Tadasana (see pages 30–31).

2 To assume Paschima Namaskar, or Reverse Prayer, bring your hands together behind your back. Bend your knees slightly, and round your torso forward. Touch your fingertips together, and rotate them inward toward the center of your shoulder blades. Once your fingers are pointing upward with your hands parallel to your spine, stand up tall, and draw your elbows forward, keeping your shoulders down.

3 Exhale, and take one large step forward with your right leg. Turn your back foot out slightly, and keep your right foot pointed forward. Square your hips forward by rotating your torso slightly to the right, and tuck your tailbone toward your pubis. Press your left heel to the floor, and contract your leg muscles. Lift up tall through your spine and chest.

4 Exhale, and begin to lean your torso forward, making sure to keep your back flat. Stretch forward until your torso is parallel to the floor. Make sure your leg muscles are still contracted and your feet firmly grounded.

5 With your back flat, draw your torso down to your right thigh.

6 Hold for 15 to 30 seconds. Repeat with your left leg in front.

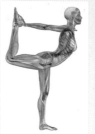

PRIMARY TARGETS
- biceps femoris
- semitendinosus
- gluteus medius
- gluteus maximus
- gastrocnemius
- soleus
- deltoideus

BENEFITS
- Stretches spine, shoulders, and hamstrings
- Strengthens legs
- Stimulates digestion

CAUTIONS
- High blood pressure
- Back injury

PERFECT YOUR FORM
- Keep your back heel on the floor.
- Avoid rounding your spine to lower your torso to your front leg.
- Avoid turning your hips out to either side.
- If your shoulders aren't flexible enough to do this pose in Paschima Namaskar, place your hands on the floor or bend your arms behind your back and cross them, holding each elbow in your opposite hand.

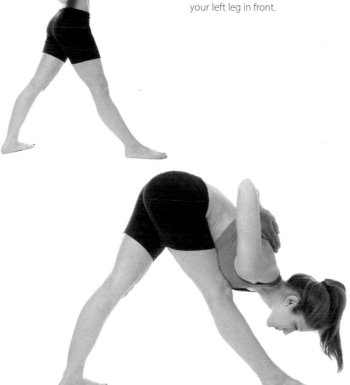

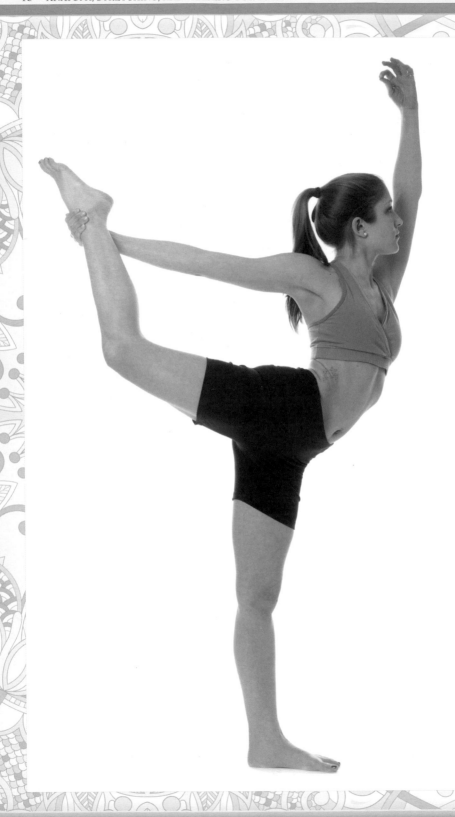

YOGA BACKBENDS

Yoga novices often view back-bending asanas as unfamiliar and uncomfortable—and reasonably so. Many of us spend much of our lives bending forward or hunched over in chairs. The benefits of the back-bending poses, however, go far beyond simply improving posture. Backbends are more like full-body bends. They will stretch your shoulders, abdominals, and tops of your legs, and they will open your chest, strengthen your back, and create mobility in your hips and spine. They are invigorating and build a healthy nervous system.

It is important when entering back-bending poses that you exercise a great deal of patience. Go slowly and carefully, and do not force your body into a deeper or a more advanced pose than your muscles are ready for. Make sure that you have warmed up properly, and take special precaution if you have a chronic or recent back injury.

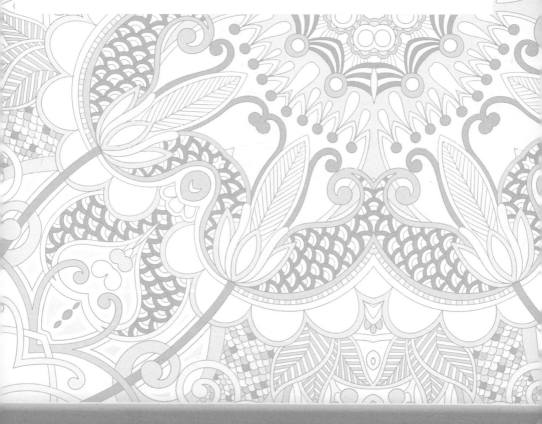

MARJARYASANA TO BITILASANA

BEGINNER

(Cat Pose to Cow Pose; Cat-Cow)

MARJARYASANA TO BITILASANA—Cat Pose to Cow Pose, or more simply, Cat-Cow—combines two yoga asanas to create a flow of breath-synchronized movement. Start off your yoga session with a few repetitions of Cat-Cow to warm up your spine and release any residual tension of the day.

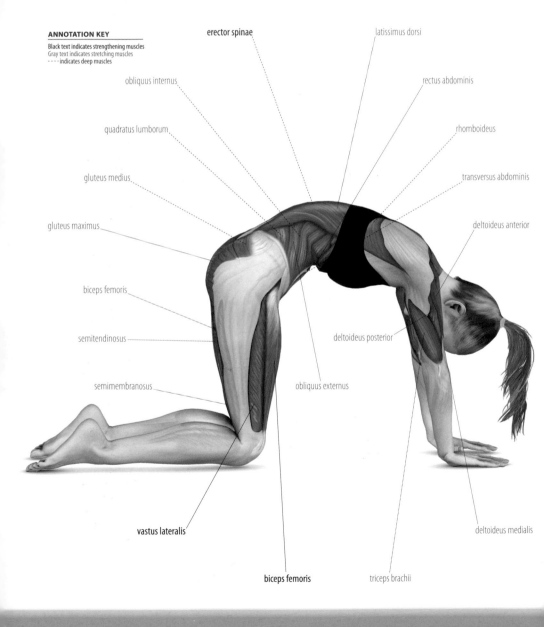

ANNOTATION KEY
Black text indicates strengthening muscles
Gray text indicates stretching muscles
----indicates deep muscles

erector spinae

latissimus dorsi

obliquus internus

rectus abdominis

quadratus lumborum

rhomboideus

gluteus medius

transversus abdominis

gluteus maximus

deltoideus anterior

biceps femoris

semitendinosus

deltoideus posterior

semimembranosus

obliquus externus

vastus lateralis

deltoideus medialis

biceps femoris

triceps brachii

HOW TO DO IT

1 Begin on your hands and knees, with your wrists directly below your shoulders and your knees directly below your hips. Your fingertips should be facing forward with your hands one shoulder-width apart. Gaze at the floor, keeping your head in a neutral position.

2 Exhale, and round your spine up toward the ceiling, dropping your head. Draw your abdominals in toward your spine. Keep your hips lifted and your shoulders in the same position.

3 Inhale, and uncurl your spine. Remain on your hands and knees.

4 With your next inhalation, arch your spine, lifting your chest forward and your sit bones up toward the ceiling. Gaze forward.

5 Exhale, and return to a neutral position on your hands and knees.

6 Repeat Marjaryasana to Bitilasana 10 to 20 times.

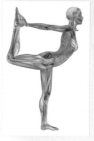

PRIMARY TARGETS
- erector spinae
- latissimus dorsi
- obliquus externus
- obliquus internus
- rectus abdominis

BENEFITS
- Stretches chest, shoulders, neck, spine, and abdominals
- Improves range of motion

CAUTIONS
- Knee injury
- Wrist pain

PERFECT YOUR FORM
- Stretch slowly and with control.
- Keep your hands and feet firmly planted throughout the stretch.
- Lift your chin while your spine is arched.
- Start the movement of your spine in your tailbone.
- Draw your shoulders away from your neck.
- Avoid arching, primarily in your lower back.
- Avoid tucking your chin to your chest in Marjaryasana.
- Avoid jutting your ribs out in Bitilasana.

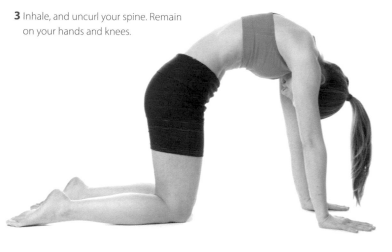

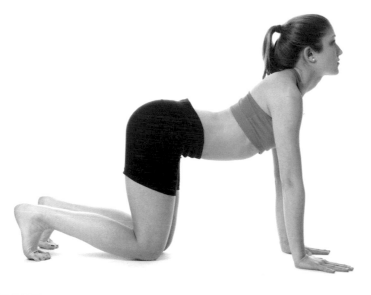

BHUJANGASANA

BEGINNER

(Cobra Pose)

BHUJANGASANA, or Cobra Pose, takes its name from the raised-hood stance of a cobra about to strike. When you properly execute this asana, your body will take on the raised-hood position. It is a rejuvenating pose and slowly stretches your entire spinal column and the muscles surrounding it, as well as stretches your glutes, chest, and abdominals.

ANNOTATION KEY

Black text indicates strengthening muscles
Gray text indicates stretching muscles
----indicates deep muscles

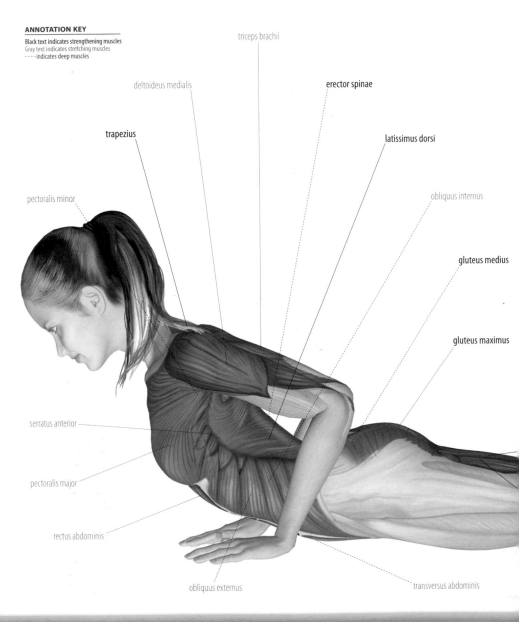

triceps brachii

deltoideus medialis

erector spinae

trapezius

latissimus dorsi

pectoralis minor

obliquus internus

gluteus medius

gluteus maximus

serratus anterior

pectoralis major

rectus abdominis

obliquus externus

transversus abdominis

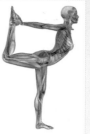

YOGA BACKBENDS

HOW TO DO IT

1 Lie prone on the floor. Bend your elbows, placing your hands flat on the floor beside your chest. Keep your elbows pulled in toward your body. Extend your legs, pressing your pubis, thighs, and tops of your feet into the floor.

2 Inhale, and lift your chest off the floor, pushing down with your hands to guide your lift. Keep your pubis pressed against the floor.

3 Lift through the top of your chest. Pull your tailbone down toward your pubis. Push your shoulders down and back, and elongate your neck as you gaze slightly upward.

4 Hold for 15 to 30 seconds, and exhale as you lower yourself to the floor.

PRIMARY TARGETS
- quadratus lumborum
- erector spinae
- latissimus dorsi
- gluteus maximus
- gluteus medius
- pectoralis major
- rectus abdominis
- deltoideus
- teres major
- teres minor

BENEFITS
- Strengthens spine and buttocks
- Stretches chest, abdominals, and shoulders

CAUTIONS
- Back injury

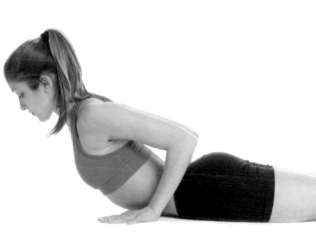

PERFECT YOUR FORM
- Lift out of your chest and back, rather than depend too much on your arms to create the arch in your back.
- Keep your shoulders and elbows pressed back to create more lift in your chest.
- Don't tense your buttocks, which adds pressure on your lower back.
- Avoid lifting your hips off the floor.

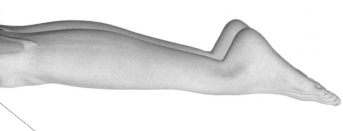

biceps femoris

semitendinosus

URDHVA MUKHA SVANASANA

(Upward-Facing Dog Pose)

URDHVA MUKHA SVANASANA, or Upward-Facing Dog, is one of the positions in the Sun Salutation sequences and is also performed in many yoga flow classes. A resting asana, it is similar to Bhujangasana, stretching your glutes, chest, and abdominals. More active than Bhujangasana, it tones and strengthens your quadriceps and lower back.

ANNOTATION KEY
Black text indicates strengthening muscles
Gray text indicates stretching muscles
- - - - indicates deep muscles

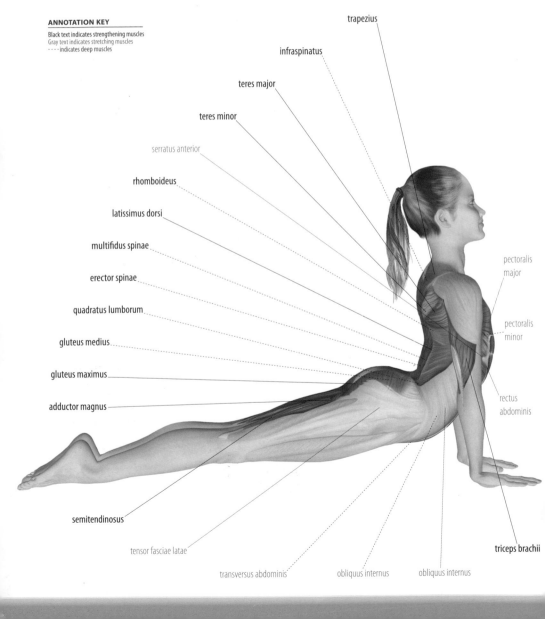

trapezius

infraspinatus

teres major

teres minor

serratus anterior

rhomboideus

latissimus dorsi

multifidus spinae

erector spinae

quadratus lumborum

gluteus medius

gluteus maximus

adductor magnus

pectoralis major

pectoralis minor

rectus abdominis

semitendinosus

tensor fasciae latae

transversus abdominis

obliquus internus

obliquus internus

triceps brachii

HOW TO DO IT

1 Lie prone on the floor. Bend your elbows, placing your hands flat on the floor on either side of your chest. Keep your elbows pulled in toward your body. Separate your legs one hip-width apart, and extend through your toes. The tops of your feet should be touching the floor.

2 Inhale, and press against the floor with your hands and the tops of your feet, lifting your torso and hips off the floor.

Contract your thighs, and tuck your tailbone toward your pubis.

3 Lift through the top of your chest, fully extending your arms and creating an arch in your back from your upper torso. Push your shoulders down and back, and elongate your neck as you gaze slightly upward.

4 Hold for 15 to 30 seconds, and exhale as you lower yourself to the floor.

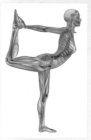

PRIMARY TARGETS
- rhomboideus
- teres major
- teres minor
- trapezius
- latissimus dorsi
- erector spinae
- quadratus lumborum
- gluteus maximus
- pectoralis major
- serratus anterior
- rectus abdominis
- triceps brachii

BENEFITS
- Strengthens spine, arms, and wrists
- Stretches chest and abdominals
- Improves posture

CAUTIONS
- Back injury
- Wrist injury or carpal tunnel syndrome

PERFECT YOUR FORM
- Elongate your legs and arms to create full extension.
- Make sure that your wrists are positioned directly below your shoulders so that you don't exert too much pressure on your lower back.

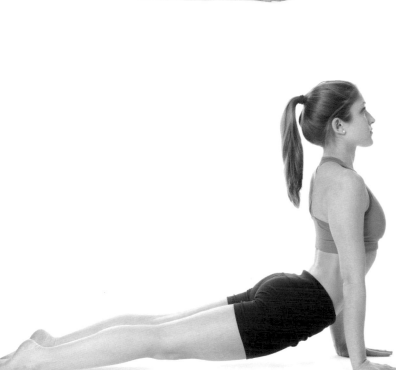

SALABHASANA

BEGINNER

(Locust Pose; Grasshopper Pose)

WITH MANY OF THE SAME BENEFITS as Bhujangasana and Urdhva Mukha Svanasana, Salabhasana is a mild backbend that strengthens your upper and lower back, arms, and legs while stretching your chest, shoulders, and abdominals. Practicing Salabhasana, also known as Locust Pose or Grasshopper Pose, will prepare your body for deeper backbends.

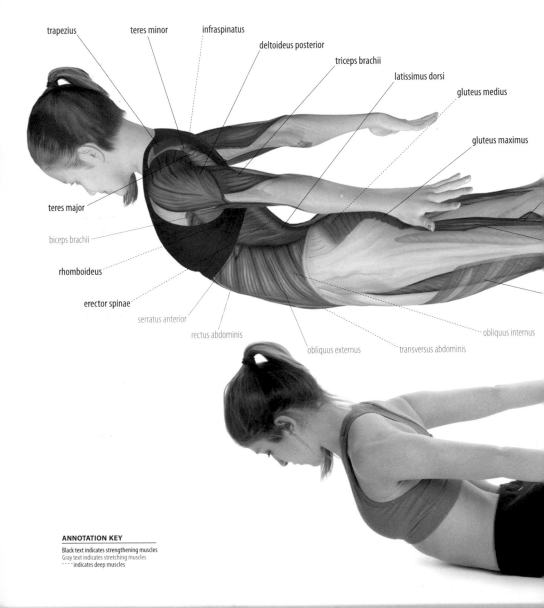

trapezius

teres minor

infraspinatus

deltoideus posterior

triceps brachii

latissimus dorsi

gluteus medius

gluteus maximus

teres major

biceps brachii

rhomboideus

erector spinae

serratus anterior

rectus abdominis

obliquus externus

transversus abdominis

obliquus internus

ANNOTATION KEY

Black text indicates strengthening muscles
Gray text indicates stretching muscles
- - - indicates deep muscles

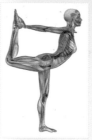

HOW TO DO IT

1 Lie prone on the floor with your arms resting by your sides and the palms of your hands facing downward. Turn your legs in toward each other so that your knees point directly into the floor.

legs behind you, with your arms parallel to the floor. Lift up as high as possible, with your pelvis and lower abdominals stabilizing your body on the floor. Keep your head in a neutral position.

2 Squeezing your buttocks, inhale, and lift up your head, chest, arms, and legs simultaneously. Extend your arms and

3 Hold for 30 seconds to 1 minute. Repeat 1 to 2 times.

PRIMARY TARGETS
- rhomboideus
- infraspinatus
- teres major
- latissimus dorsi
- deltoideus
- erector spinae
- trapezius
- gluteus maximus
- gluteus medius

BENEFITS
- Strengthens spine, buttocks, arms, and legs
- Stretches hip flexors, chest, and abdominals
- Stimulates digestion

CAUTIONS
- Back injury

PERFECT YOUR FORM
- Elongate the back of your neck.
- Open your chest to extend the arch through your entire spine.
- Avoid bending your knees.
- Don't hold your breath.

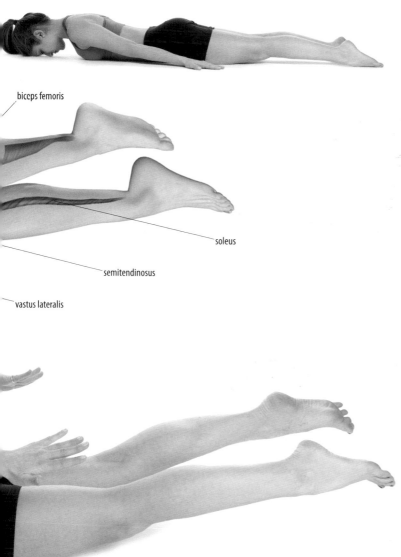

biceps femoris

soleus

semitendinosus

vastus lateralis

MATSYASANA

BEGINNER

(Fish Pose)

MATSYASANA, OR FISH POSE, is one of the basic poses of both Ashtanga and Hatha yoga. It works wells as a counterpose to shoulderstands, opening your pectoral muscles, the intercostal muscles between your ribs, and the iliopsoas muscles of your hips. Proper form calls for you to take deep inhalations, resting the weight of your body on your hips and elbows while your head rests gently on the floor.

ANNOTATION KEY

Black text indicates strengthening muscles
Gray text indicates stretching muscles
----indicates deep muscles

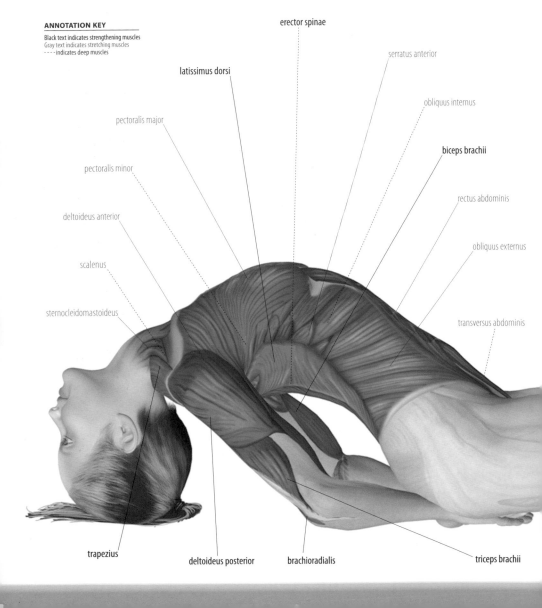

erector spinae

serratus anterior

obliquus internus

latissimus dorsi

biceps brachii

pectoralis major

rectus abdominis

pectoralis minor

obliquus externus

deltoideus anterior

scalenus

sternocleidomastoideus

transversus abdominis

trapezius

deltoideus posterior

brachioradialis

triceps brachii

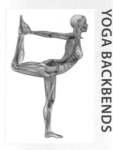

HOW TO DO IT

1 Lie supine on the floor with your arms by your sides. Push down into your heels to lift your hips, and place your hands beneath your buttocks, with your palms facing down.

2 Rest your buttocks on the tops of your hands, and elongate your legs. Inhale, and press down with your forearms, slightly bending your elbows. Lift your chest and head off the floor, creating an arch in your upper back.

3 Tilt your head back, and place it on the floor. Keep the majority of your weight on your elbows.

4 Hold for 15 to 30 seconds.

PRIMARY TARGETS
- rhomboideus
- teres major
- teres minor
- latissimus dorsi
- trapezius
- pectoralis major
- deltoideus anterior
- sternocleidomastoideus
- serratus anterior

BENEFITS
- Stretches chest and abdominals
- Strengthens neck, shoulders, and spine
- Improves posture

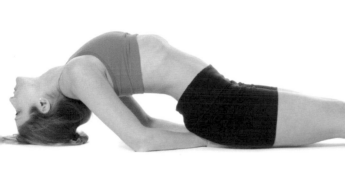

CAUTIONS
- Back injury
- High or low blood pressure
- Headache

PERFECT YOUR FORM
- Avoid pushing your weight onto your head and neck.

SETU BANDHASANA

BEGINNER
(Bridge Pose; Spinal Lift Pose)

SETU BANDHASANA, most commonly known as Bridge Pose, awakens both your body and mind. While preparing you for more challenging backbends, this exhilarating asana will open your chest and stretch your spine, as well as tone your quadriceps and glutes.

ANNOTATION KEY
Black text indicates strengthening muscles
Gray text indicates stretching muscles
----indicates deep muscles

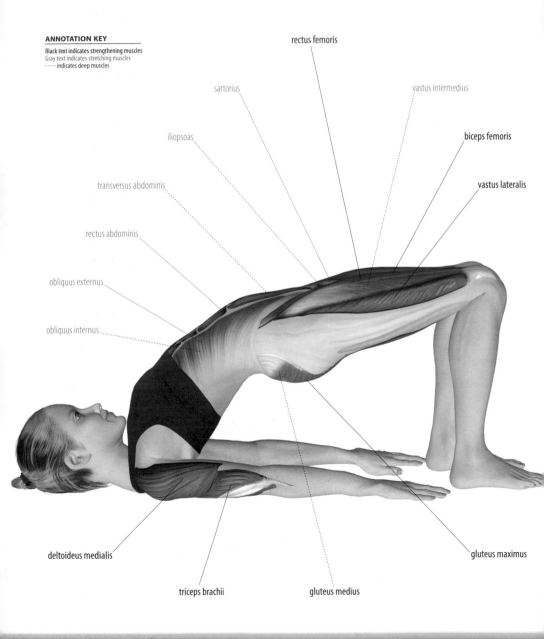

rectus femoris

sartorius

vastus intermedius

iliopsoas

biceps femoris

transversus abdominis

vastus lateralis

rectus abdominis

obliquus externus

obliquus internus

deltoideus medialis

gluteus maximus

triceps brachii

gluteus medius

HOW TO DO IT

1 Lie supine on the floor. Bend your knees and draw you heels close to your buttocks. Place you hands flat on the floor by your sides.

2 Exhale, and press down though your feet to lift your buttocks off the floor. With your feet and thighs parallel, push your arms into the floor while extending through your fingertips.

3 Lengthen your neck away from your shoulders. Lift your hips higher so that your torso rises from the floor.

4 Hold for 30 seconds to 1 minute. Exhale as you release your spine onto the floor, one vertebra at a time. Repeat at least one more time.

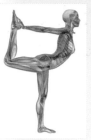

PRIMARY TARGETS
- sartorius
- rectus femoris
- iliopsoas
- gluteus maximus
- gluteus medius
- erector spinae

BENEFITS
- Strengthens thighs and buttocks
- Stretches chest and spine
- Stimulates digestion
- Stimulates thyroid
- Reduces stress

CAUTIONS
- Shoulder injury
- Back injury
- Neck issues

PERFECT YOUR FORM
- Keep your knees over your heels.

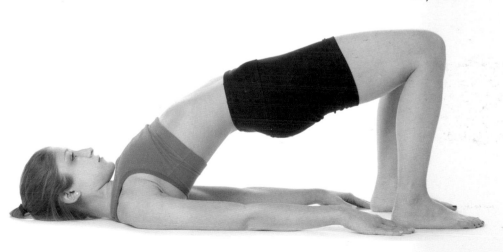

SUPTA VIRASANA

INTERMEDIATE

(Reclining Hero Pose)

Supta Virasana, or Reclining Hero Pose, is a challenging version of the upright Virasana (see page 21). In Supta Virasana, you recline your body backward, intensifying the stretch in your thighs, groins, knees, ankles, and abdomen. This passive and restorative backbend opens your chest and is a wonderful way to counteract the forward rounding of the back that results from days spent sitting at a desk.

ANNOTATION KEY
Black text indicates strengthening muscles
Gray text indicates stretching muscles
- - - - indicates deep muscles

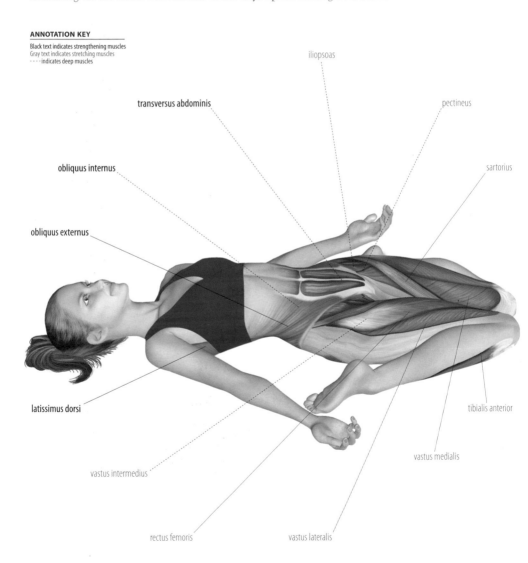

iliopsoas

transversus abdominis

pectineus

obliquus internus

sartorius

obliquus externus

latissimus dorsi

tibialis anterior

vastus medialis

vastus intermedius

rectus femoris

vastus lateralis

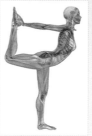

HOW TO DO IT

1 Begin by sitting in Virasana (see page 21). Make sure that you are comfortable sitting with your buttocks completely on the floor.

2 Lean back gradually, and exhale, placing your hands on the floor behind you for support. Carefully lower yourself onto your elbows.

3 Recline all the way until your back reaches the floor. Move your arms to your sides, relaxing them with your palms facing upward. Squeeze your knees together so they don't separate wider than your hips, and don't allow them to lift off the floor.

4 Hold for 30 seconds to 1 minute.

PRIMARY TARGETS
- iliopsoas
- pectineus
- sartorius
- biceps femoris
- vastus intermedius
- vastus medialis
- tibialis anterior
- rectus femoris

BENEFITS
- Loosens thighs, knees, hip flexors, and ankles
- Stimulates digestion
- Alleviates arthritis
- Alleviates respiratory problems

CAUTIONS
- Knee injury
- Ankle injury
- Back issues

PERFECT YOUR FORM
- Avoid sliding your knees beyond the width of your hips.

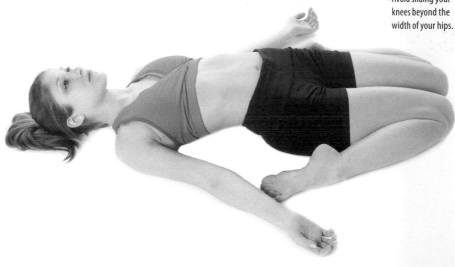

ARDHA BHEKASANA

INTERMEDIATE

(Half-Frog Pose)

ARDHA BHEKASANA, or Half-Frog Pose, stretches your quadriceps, abdominals, and shoulders while opening your chest and upper back. If you're a runner, Ardha Bhekasana works well as an alternate prerun quad stretch. It is a challenging asana, so be careful to not push too hard on your foot if you feel any pain in your knee.

ANNOTATION KEY
Black text indicates strengthening muscles
Gray text indicates stretching muscles
- - - -indicates deep muscles

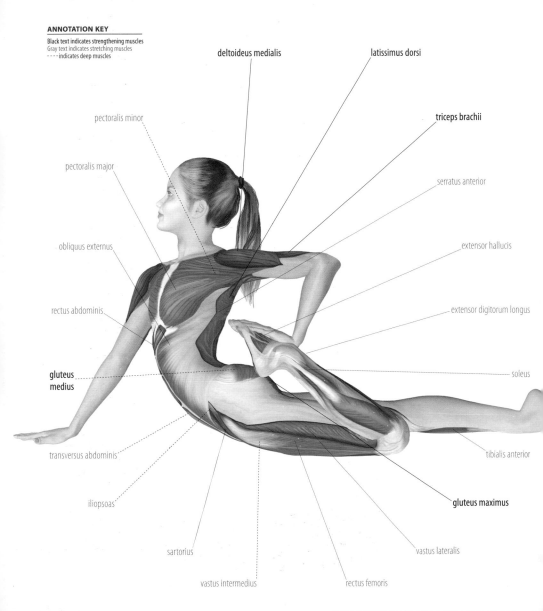

deltoideus medialis

latissimus dorsi

pectoralis minor

triceps brachii

pectoralis major

serratus anterior

obliquus externus

extensor hallucis

rectus abdominis

extensor digitorum longus

gluteus medius

soleus

transversus abdominis

iliopsoas

gluteus maximus

tibialis anterior

sartorius

vastus lateralis

vastus intermedius

rectus femoris

HOW TO DO IT

1 Lie prone on the floor with your legs fully extended. Bend your elbows, placing your hands flat on the floor on either side of your chest. Keep your elbows pulled in toward your body.

2 Inhale, and press into the floor with your hands, lifting your chest and upper torso off the floor. Push your shoulders down and back. Keep your pubis pressed against the floor. Your hands should be placed slightly in front of your torso.

3 Bend your left knee, drawing your left heel toward your left buttock. Shift your weight onto your right hand, and reach behind you with your left hand to grasp the inside of your left foot. Continue to lift your chest and push down with your right shoulder.

4 Bend your left elbow up toward the ceiling, and rotate your hand so that it rests on top of your foot with your fingers facing forward. Exhale, and press down on your foot with your left hand to stretch it toward your left buttock.

5 Without separating your legs more than one hip-width apart, deepen the stretch by moving your left foot slightly to the outside of your left thigh, aiming the sole of your foot toward the floor.

6 Hold for 30 seconds to 2 minutes. Repeat on the opposite side.

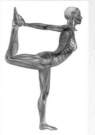

PRIMARY TARGETS
- latissimus dorsi
- quadratus lumborum
- erector spinae
- pectoralis major
- deltoideus medialis
- rectus abdominis
- transversus abdominis
- iliopsoas
- vastus intermedius
- rectus femoris
- sartorius
- tibialis anterior
- extensor hallucis

BENEFITS
- Strengthens spine and shoulders
- Stretches chest, abdominals, hip flexors, quadriceps, and ankles

CAUTIONS
- High or low blood pressure
- Back injury
- Shoulder injury

PERFECT YOUR FORM
- If you have trouble supporting yourself on your hand, lower yourself onto your forearm and elbow.

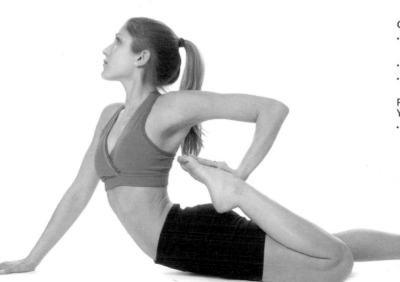

DHANURASANA

(Bow Pose)

COMBINING THE BENEFITS of Bhujangasana and Salabhasana, Dhanurasana, or Bow Pose, strengthens the arms, legs, abdomen, and spine. A basic posture of Hatha yoga, you'll find this energy-boosting asana included in many classes. Its full backward bend builds spinal strength and flexibility, and it works as a counterpose to forward bends.

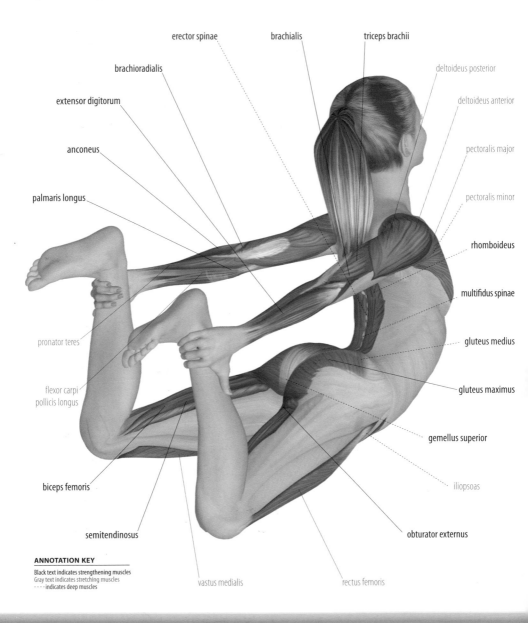

erector spinae
brachialis
triceps brachii
deltoideus posterior
brachioradialis
deltoideus anterior
extensor digitorum
pectoralis major
anconeus
pectoralis minor
palmaris longus
rhomboideus
multifidus spinae
gluteus medius
pronator teres
gluteus maximus
flexor carpi pollicis longus
gemellus superior
iliopsoas
biceps femoris
obturator externus
semitendinosus

ANNOTATION KEY
Black text indicates strengthening muscles
Gray text indicates stretching muscles
----indicates deep muscles

vastus medialis
rectus femoris

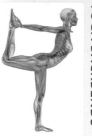

HOW TO DO IT

1 Lie prone on the floor, and place your arms by your sides with your palms facing upward.

2 Place your chin on the floor, and exhale as you bend your knees. Reach your arms behind you, and grasp the outside of your ankles with your hands.

3 Inhale, and lift your chest off the floor. Simultaneously lift your thighs by pulling your ankles up with your hands. Shift your weight onto your abdominals.

4 Keep your head in a neutral position, and make sure that your knees don't separate more than the width of your hips. Tuck your tailbone into your pubis.

5 Hold for 20 to 30 seconds. Exhale, and release your ankles, gently returning to the floor.

PRIMARY TARGETS
- pectoralis major
- pectoralis minor
- deltoideus anterior
- deltoideus posterior
- erector spinae
- gluteus medius
- gluteus maximus
- iliopsoas
- rectus femoris

BENEFITS
- Strengthens spine
- Stretches chest, abdominals, hip flexors, and quadriceps
- Stimulates digestion

CAUTIONS
- Headache
- High or low blood pressure
- Back injury

PERFECT YOUR FORM
- Keep your knees close together during the duration of the posture, making sure that they don't separate more than the width of your hips.
- Breathing in this pose can be difficult, so make sure to take short, controlled breaths from the back of your torso.
- Avoid rolling back onto your pelvis to support your weight.

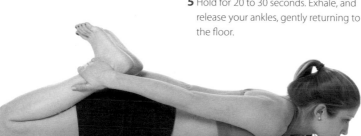

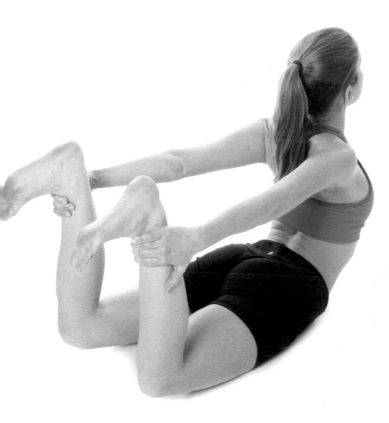

URDHVA DHANURASANA

INTERMEDIATE

(Wheel Pose; Upward-Facing Bow Pose)

URDHVA DHANURASANA, also known as Upward Bow Pose or Wheel Pose, is a physically challenging pose, but it is also an uplifting posture that stimulates your energy and vitality. This full backbend improves spinal flexibility, stretches your chest and shoulder muscles, and strengthens your arms, legs, abdomen, and spine. When practicing Urdhva Dhanurasana aim for steadiness of both mind and body.

ANNOTATION KEY
Black text indicates strengthening muscles
Gray text indicates stretching muscles
- - - - indicates deep muscles

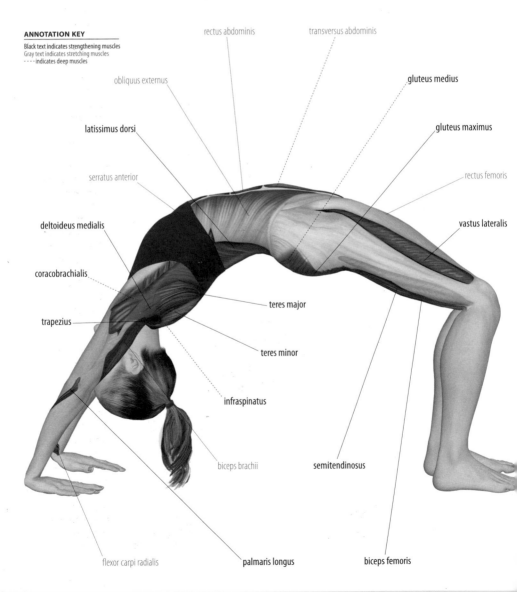

rectus abdominis

transversus abdominis

obliquus externus

gluteus medius

gluteus maximus

latissimus dorsi

rectus femoris

serratus anterior

deltoideus medialis

vastus lateralis

coracobrachialis

teres major

trapezius

teres minor

infraspinatus

biceps brachii

semitendinosus

flexor carpi radialis

palmaris longus

biceps femoris

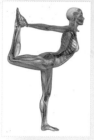

HOW TO DO IT

1 Lie supine on the floor. Bend your knees, and draw your heels as close to your buttocks as possible. Bend your elbows, and place your hands on the floor beside your head, with your fingertips pointing toward your shoulders.

2 Exhale, and push down into your feet to lift your buttocks off the floor. Tighten your thighs, and keep your feet parallel. Push your hands into the floor to raise yourself onto the crown of your head.

3 After a couple of breaths, exhale, and press into the floor with your hands

and feet, lifting your hips up toward the ceiling. Straighten your arms, and allow your head to hang in between your shoulders. Push through your legs, straightening them as much as possible. Open your shoulders, and feel the extension through your entire spine.

4 Hold for 5 to 30 seconds. Exhale as you bend your arms, and slowly lower yourself to the floor. Repeat at least 1 time.

PRIMARY TARGETS
- deltoideus medialis
- serratus anterior
- infraspinatus
- rhomboideus
- flexor carpi radialis
- latissimus dorsi
- trapezius
- erector spinae
- gluteus maximus
- vastus lateralis
- teres major
- teres minor

BENEFITS
- Strengthens thighs and buttocks
- Stretches chest and spine
- Stimulates digestion
- Stimulates thyroid
- Reduces stress

CAUTIONS
- Back injury
- Carpal tunnel syndrome
- High or low blood pressure
- Headache

PERFECT YOUR FORM
- Lift up, and extend through your shoulders, spine, and quadriceps, being careful not to put all the extension on your lower back.
- Keep your knees separated no wider than the width of your hips.

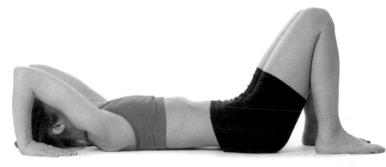

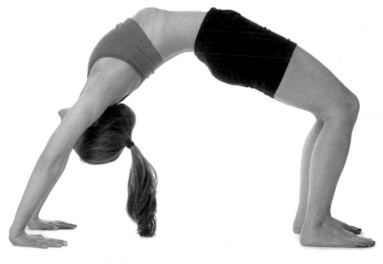

UTRASANA

INTERMEDIATE

(Camel Pose)

UTRASANA, OR CAMEL POSE, stretches nearly all the major muscles of your body, while also toning your chest, abdomen, and thighs. Practice this backbend when your back is fully warmed up, and be sure to slowly enter the pose to avoid feeling light-headed. If you find the pose hard on your knees, place a folded blanket or other padding beneath them.

ANNOTATION KEY

Black text indicates strengthening muscles
Gray text indicates stretching muscles
----indicates deep muscles

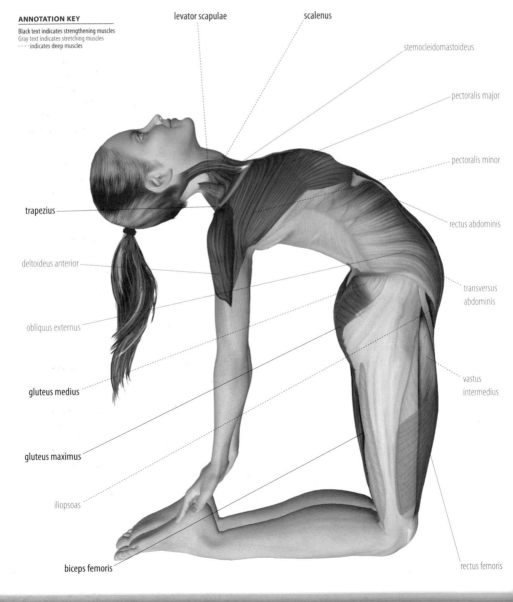

levator scapulae

scalenus

sternocleidomastoideus

pectoralis major

pectoralis minor

rectus abdominis

trapezius

deltoideus anterior

obliquus externus

transversus abdominis

gluteus medius

vastus intermedius

gluteus maximus

iliopsoas

biceps femoris

rectus femoris

HOW TO DO IT

1 With your knees one hip-width apart, kneel on the floor with your thighs perpendicular to the floor and your hips open. Tuck your tailbone toward your pubis, and lift up through your spine.

2 Place your hands on your lower back with your elbows bent and your fingers pointed toward your buttocks. Lean your shoulders and upper torso backward, opening your chest and pushing forward with your hips.

3 Exhale, and drop back, pressing your pelvis upward and elongating your spine. Pressing your shoulder blades back, lean slightly to your right, and

place your right hand on your right heel. Lean slightly to your left, and place your left hand on your left heel. Your fingers should be pointed toward your toes.

4 Push your thighs forward and center your weight in between your knees, lifting your chest into the arch. Drop your head back, and relax your throat.

5 Hold for 20 seconds to 1 minute. To come out of the pose, contract your abdominals to lift your chest forward, and slowly bring your hands to your lower back before returning to the starting position.

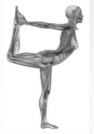

PRIMARY TARGETS
• pectoralis major
• pectoralis minor
• sternocleidomastoideus
• trapezius
• rectus abdominis
• erector spinae
• gluteus medius
• gluteus maximus
• iliopsoas
• deltoideus anterior
• quadratus lumborum

BENEFITS
• Strengthens spine
• Stretches thighs, hip flexors, chest, and abdominals
• Stimulates digestion

CAUTIONS
• Back injury
• High or low blood pressure
• Headache

PERFECT YOUR FORM
• Keep your pelvis pressed forward, and lift up with your abdominals.
• Avoid compressing your lower back.
• Don't rush into the backbend, which can strain your back.

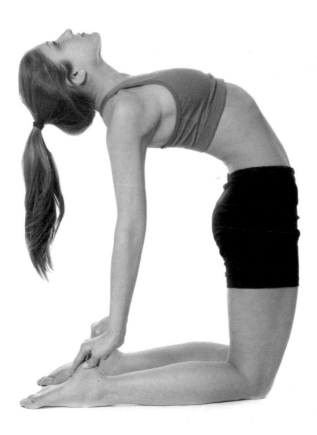

EKA PADA RAJAKAPOTASANA

ADVANCED *(Pigeon Pose; One-Legged Royal Pigeon Pose; One-Legged King Pigeon Pose; One-Footed King Pigeon Pose; King of the Pigeons Pose; Mermaid Pose)*

EKA PADA RAJAKAPOTASANA translates from the Sanskrit as "One-Legged Royal Pigeon Pose," and goes by many variations of that name because the backbend puffs up your chest making you resemble a pigeon. Also known as Mermaid Pose, this a graceful-looking asana that opens the hips, chest, and shoulders and stretches the thighs, groins, back, gluteals, and hip flexors and extensors.

ANNOTATION KEY
Black text indicates strengthening muscles
Gray text indicates stretching muscles
- - - - indicates deep muscles

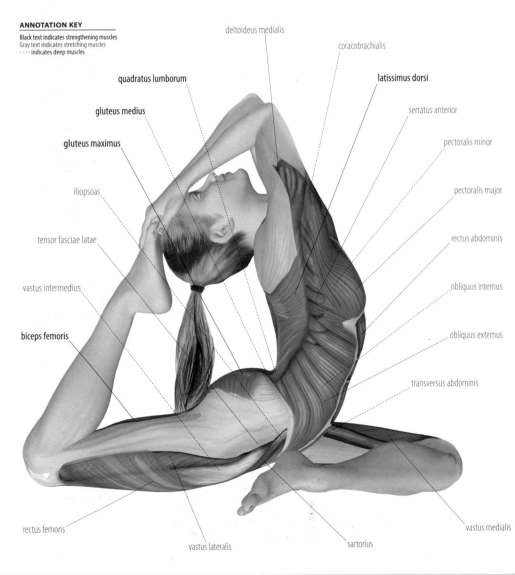

deltoideus medialis

coracobrachialis

quadratus lumborum

latissimus dorsi

gluteus medius

serratus anterior

gluteus maximus

pectoralis minor

iliopsoas

pectoralis major

tensor fasciae latae

rectus abdominis

vastus intermedius

obliquus internus

biceps femoris

obliquus externus

transversus abdominis

rectus femoris

vastus medialis

vastus lateralis

sartorius

HOW TO DO IT

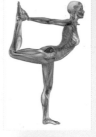

1 Begin in Adho Mukha Svanasana (see page 22). Bend your left knee, and bring it forward, in between your hands. Place your left leg on the floor with your knee still bent, lowering your shin and thigh to the floor. Your left heel should point toward your pubis.

2 Extend your right leg behind you. Your hips should be squared forward, and your right knee should point down toward the floor.

3 Lift your chest, using your fingertips to bring your torso to an upright position. Press down into the floor with your hips and pubis, and lift up with your chest.

4 Bend your right knee, and flex your foot, drawing your heel toward your buttock. Reach back with your right hand, your palm facing up, and grasp your toes from the outside of your foot. You may keep your left fingertips on the floor in front of you for balance.

5 Point your right elbow up toward the ceiling, pull your sternum upward, and point your toes. Drop your head back, and reach your left arm over your head to grasp your toes with your left hand. Pull your foot toward your head.

6 Hold for 10 seconds to 1 minute. Return to Adho Mukha Svanasana, and repeat on the other side.

PRIMARY TARGETS
- quadratus lumborum
- latissimus dorsi
- sartorius
- vastus intermedius
- iliopsoas
- serratus anterior
- obliquus externus
- pectoralis major
- pectoralis minor
- rectus abdominis

BENEFITS
- Stretches hips, thighs, spine, chest, shoulders, neck, and abdominals
- Strengthens spine

CAUTIONS
- Hip injury
- Back injury
- Knee injury

PERFECT YOUR FORM
- Keep your hips squared forward throughout the pose.
- Sit as deeply as possible into the leg position, drawing your groins toward the floor.
- Don't compensate for tight shoulders and chest by compressing your lower back.
- Avoid rolling your back knee to either side.

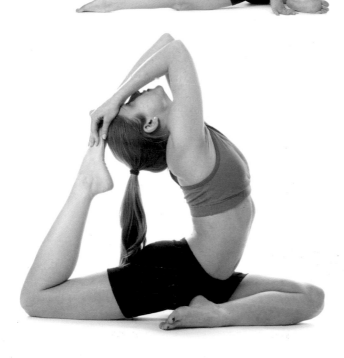

NATARAJASANA

ADVANCED

(Lord of the Dance Pose; Dancer's Pose)

NATARAJASANA, or the Lord of the Dance Pose, is a beautiful yoga asana that is also part of classical Indian dance. Its name comes from Nataraja, a depiction of the Hindu god Shiva, considered the lord of dance. Perform this full-body backbend with grace, as if you are dancing, to receive its maximum benefit.

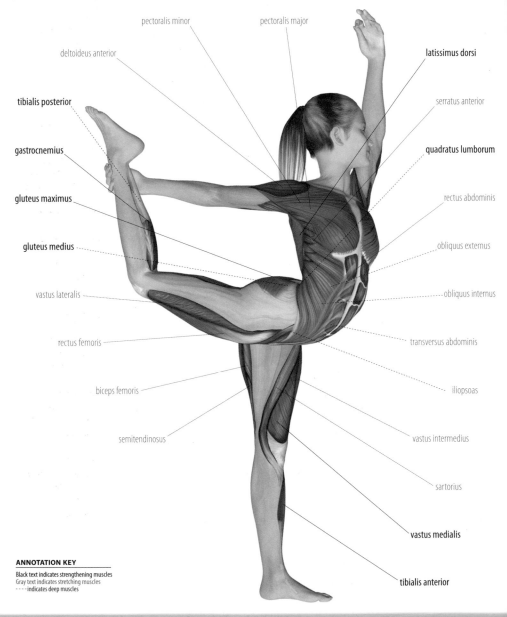

pectoralis minor

pectoralis major

deltoideus anterior

latissimus dorsi

tibialis posterior

serratus anterior

gastrocnemius

quadratus lumborum

gluteus maximus

rectus abdominis

gluteus medius

obliquus externus

vastus lateralis

obliquus internus

rectus femoris

transversus abdominis

biceps femoris

iliopsoas

semitendinosus

vastus intermedius

sartorius

vastus medialis

tibialis anterior

ANNOTATION KEY

Black text indicates strengthening muscles
Gray text indicates stretching muscles
----indicates deep muscles

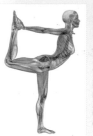

HOW TO DO IT

1 Standing in Tadasana (see pages 30–31), bend your right knee, and draw your right heel toward your buttock. Contract the muscles in your left thigh. Keep both hips open.

2 Turn your right palm outward, reach behind your back, and grasp the inside of your right foot with your hand. Lift through your spine from your tailbone to the top of your neck.

3 Raise your right foot toward the ceiling, and push back against your right hand as you lift your left arm toward the ceiling. It is natural to tilt your torso forward while raising your leg; lifting your chest and arm will help you stand upright and increase your flexibility.

4 Hold for 20 seconds to 1 minute. Release your foot and repeat on the other side.

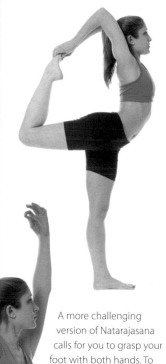

A more challenging version of Natarajasana calls for you to grasp your foot with both hands. To perform it, follow step 1. Next, turn your right palm outward, but instead of grasping the inside of your right foot, reach for the outside of your foot. Rotate your shoulder so that your right elbow points toward the ceiling. Lift your leg, and open your chest. Reach over your head with your left arm, bending your elbow to grasp your right wrist. Slowly walk your fingers back until both hands grasp your toes.

PRIMARY TARGETS
- latissimus dorsi
- pectoralis major
- pectoralis minor
- deltoideus anterior
- iliopsoas
- biceps femoris
- semitendinosus
- quadratus lumborum
- serratus anterior

BENEFITS
- Stretches thighs, groins, abdominals, shoulders, and chest
- Strengthens spine, thighs, hips, and ankles
- Improves balance

CAUTIONS
- Back injury
- Low blood pressure

PERFECT YOUR FORM
- Keep your standing leg straight and your muscles contracted.
- If you have trouble maintaining your balance, practice with your free hand against a wall for support.
- Don't look down at the floor, which may cause you to lose your balance.
- Avoid compressing your lower back.

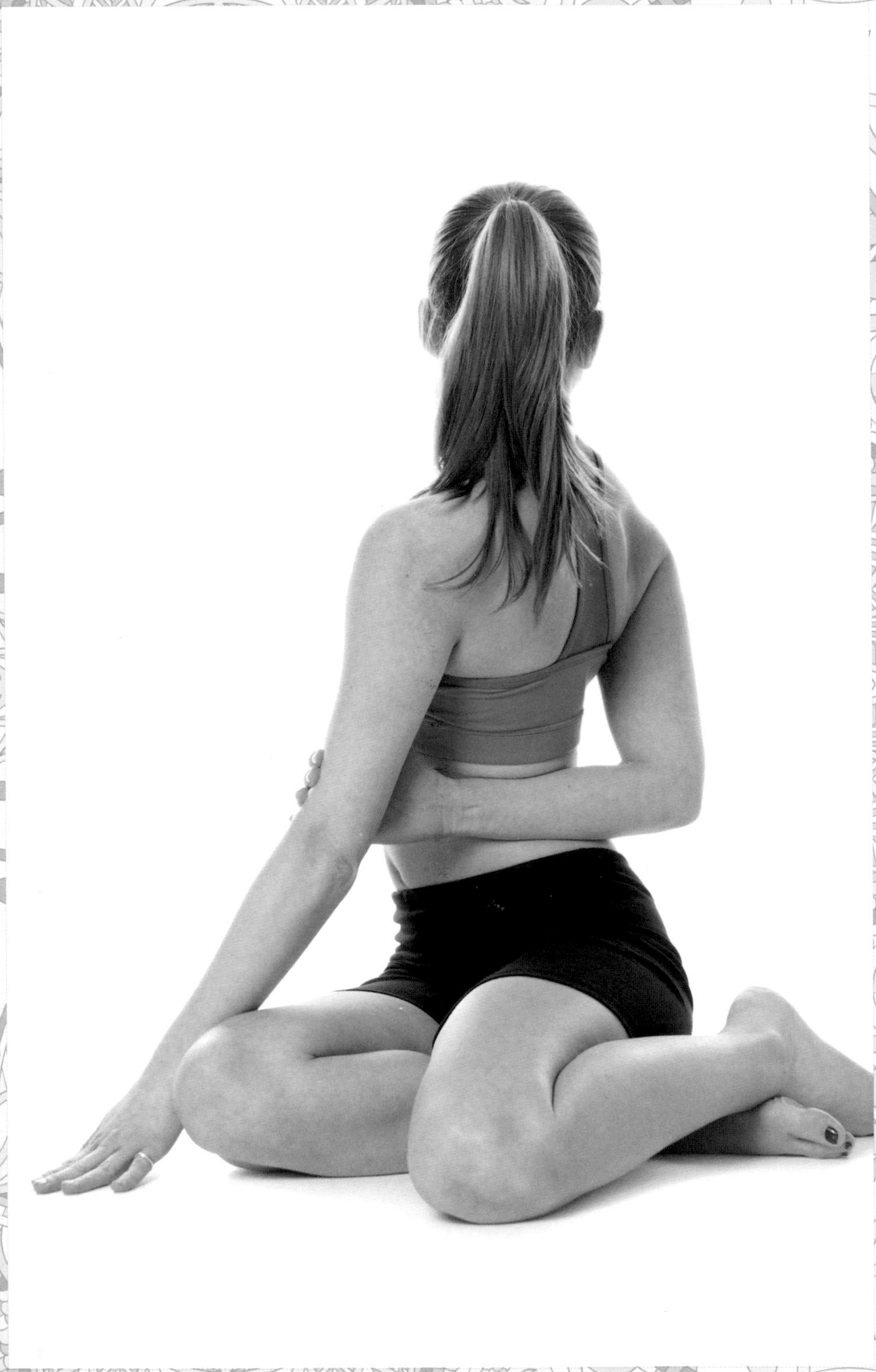

SEATED ASANAS & TWISTS

Seated and twisting asanas are refreshing poses that counteract the effects of slouching and spinal lethargy. Maintaining the proper alignment in your spine and grounding your sit bones while practicing seated poses will open your hips, groins, pelvis, and lower back. Seated poses tend to be the most stable asanas, enabling you to focus on your breath and posture.

Your muscles contract and stretch on opposite sides of your body during twisting poses. These movements target your internal organs and circulatory system, creating a cleansing effect. Your organs are compressed in the pose and refreshed upon release, and internal toxins are purged. Elongating your spine while twisting is crucial, because it will increase your spinal rotation.

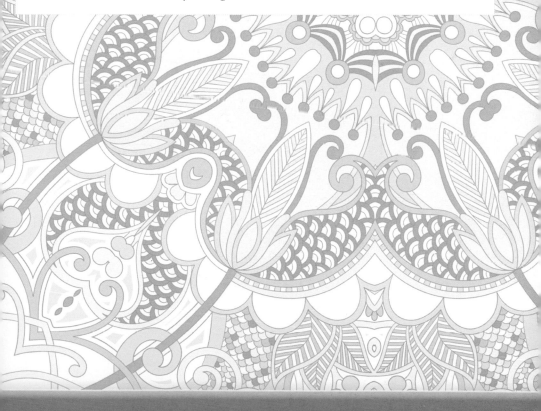

MARICHYASANA III

BEGINNER *(Marichi's Pose III; Sage Marichi Twist; Sage Twist; Ray of Light Pose)*

MARICHYASANA, or Marichi's Pose, is named for Marichi, son of the god Brahma and a sage in Indian mythology. Marichi means "ray of light," hence it is also known as Ray of Light Pose. A seated lateral twist, this asana strengthens your back and tones your abdominals.

ANNOTATION KEY
Black text indicates strengthening muscles
Gray text indicates stretching muscles
- - - - indicates deep muscles

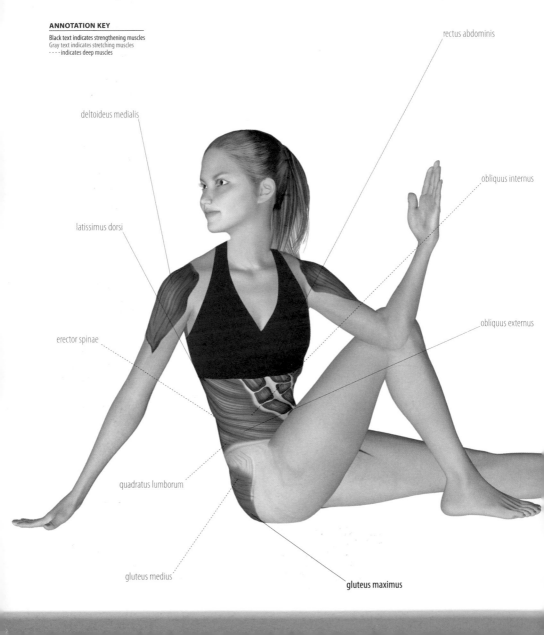

rectus abdominis

obliquus internus

deltoideus medialis

latissimus dorsi

obliquus externus

erector spinae

quadratus lumborum

gluteus medius

gluteus maximus

HOW TO DO IT

1 Sit in Dandasana (see page 19). Bend your right knee, pulling your heel toward your groin. Keep your left leg extended with your knee pointed toward the ceiling, and focus on keeping your leg grounded. Place your hands on the floor by your sides.

2 Pushing your right foot and left leg into the floor, inhale, and lift up through your spine and chest. Keep both sit bones on the floor, and relax your shoulders.

3 Exhale, and begin twisting toward your right knee. Wrap your left hand around the outside of your right thigh, pulling your knee in toward your abdominals. Press the fingertips of your right hand on the floor behind your hips. Turn your head to the right.

4 Twist deeper with each exhalation. If possible, place your left elbow on the outside of your right knee. Lean back slightly, leading with your upper torso. This will help you twist your entire spine.

5 Hold for 30 seconds to 1 minute. Gently untwist as you exhale, and repeat with your left leg bent and your right elbow over your left knee.

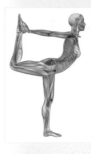

PRIMARY TARGETS
- latissimus dorsi
- multifidus spinae
- quadratus lumborum
- erector spinae
- obliquus internus
- obliquus externus
- rhomboideus

BENEFITS
- Stimulates digestion
- Strengthens and stretches spine
- Removes toxins from internal organs

CAUTIONS
- High or low blood pressure
- Back injury

PERFECT YOUR FORM
- Keep both sit bones on the floor.
- Twist from the bottom up—rotate from your lower spine, through your torso, and up through your chest.
- Avoid rounding your spine.
- Don't force a deep twist; gently ease your body into the rotation while maintaining correct upright posture.

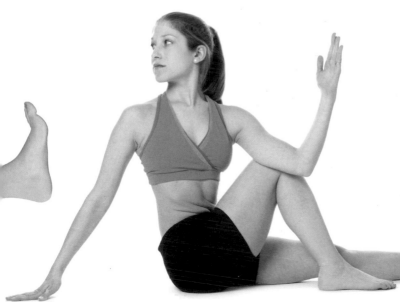

BHARADVAJASANA I

BEGINNER

(Bharadvaja's Twist)

BHARADVAJASANA I is named for an ancient Hindu seer Bharadvaja and is also called Bharadvaja's Twist. Practicing this gentle seated twist will stretch your spine, oblique muscles, torso, shoulders, and hips, leaving you feeling calm and rejuvenated.

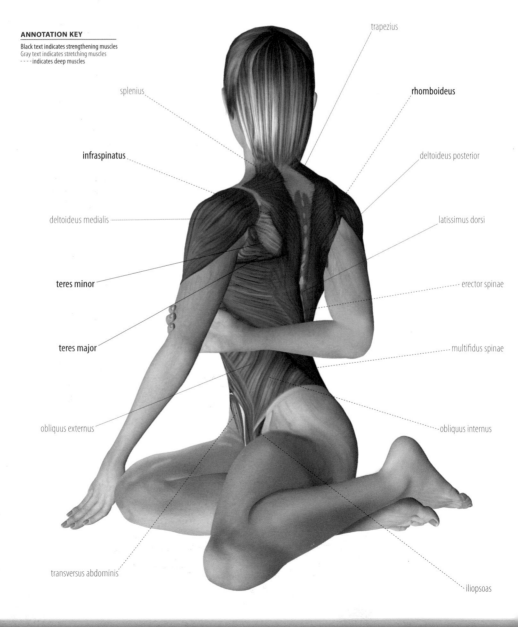

ANNOTATION KEY
Black text indicates strengthening muscles
Gray text indicates stretching muscles
- - - - indicates deep muscles

trapezius

splenius

rhomboideus

infraspinatus

deltoideus posterior

deltoideus medialis

latissimus dorsi

teres minor

erector spinae

teres major

multifidus spinae

obliquus externus

obliquus internus

transversus abdominis

iliopsoas

HOW TO DO IT

1 Sit in Dandasana (see page 19).

2 Shift your weight onto your right buttock, and bend your knees to the left, allowing your right thigh to rest on the floor. With your toes pointed toward your left hip, your left thigh should rest on top of your right calf, and your left ankle should sit on top of your right foot.

3 Inhale, and lift up from your spine. Exhale, and twist to your right, looking over your right shoulder. Place your left hand near your right knee and your right hand on the floor beside your right hip.

4 With each exhale, deepen the twist while keeping your torso upright and your shoulders pressed back. If possible, bend your right elbow, and reach across your back. Hook your right hand beneath the bend in your left elbow.

5 Hold for 30 seconds to 1 minute. Repeat on the opposite side.

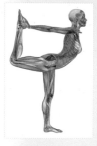

SEATED ASANAS & TWISTS

PRIMARY TARGETS
• deltoideus posterior
• rhomboideus
• latissimus dorsi
• infraspinatus
• teres major
• teres minor
• erector spinae
• multifidus spinae
• obliquus internus
• obliquus externus

BENEFITS
• Stretches spine, shoulders, and hips
• Stimulates digestion
• Relieves stress

CAUTIONS
• Low or high blood pressure
• Diarrhea

PERFECT YOUR FORM
• Try to press both sit bones into the floor while twisting.
• Avoid popping your rib cage out.
• Avoid dropping your head.

JATHARA PARIVARTANASANA

BEGINNER

*(Reclining Twist; Revolved Abdomen Pose;
Belly Twist; Belly Turning Pose)*

JATHARA PARIVARTANASANA—also known as Reclining Twist, Revolved Abdomen Pose, Belly Twist, and Belly Turning Pose—is a gentle supine twist that stretches your hips and spine while toning your abdominal muscles. Performing this asana regularly helps relieve lower-back pain and tension.

ANNOTATION KEY
Black text indicates strengthening muscles
Gray text indicates stretching muscles
- - - - indicates deep muscles

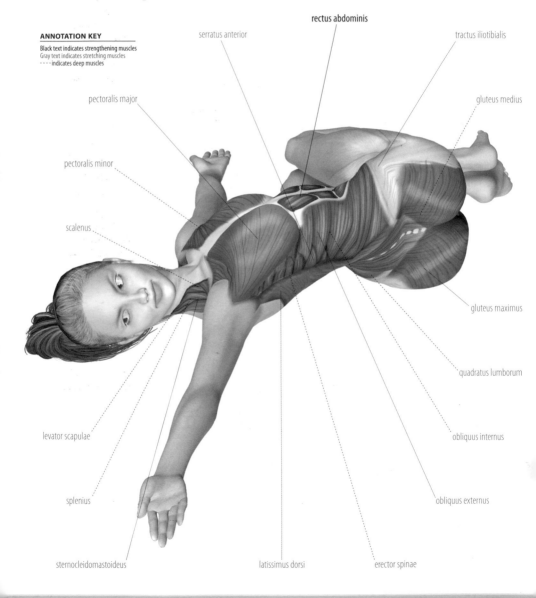

rectus abdominis

serratus anterior

tractus iliotibialis

pectoralis major

gluteus medius

pectoralis minor

scalenus

gluteus maximus

quadratus lumborum

levator scapulae

obliquus internus

splenius

obliquus externus

sternocleidomastoideus

latissimus dorsi

erector spinae

HOW TO DO IT

1 Lie on the floor in Savasana (see page 27). Bend your knees with your feet flat on the floor. Extend your arms straight out to the sides, palms facing up.

2 Inhale, and elongate your spine from your hips to the top of your neck. Lift your hips up slightly, and place them on the floor closer to your heels to lengthen and relax your spine further.

3 Lift your feet off the floor, keeping your knees bent.

4 Exhale, and bend your knees to the left, causing your hips and spine to twist. Keep your shoulder blades planted on the floor, and allow gravity to pull your left thigh to the floor with each exhalation. Turn your head to the right.

5 Hold for 30 seconds to 3 minutes. Repeat on the opposite side.

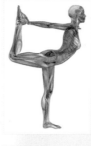

PRIMARY TARGETS
• serratus anterior
• obliquus internus
• obliquus externus
• latissimus dorsi
• erector spinae
• quadratus lumborum
• tractus iliotibialis

BENEFITS
• Releases spinal tension
• Loosens hips
• Tones abdominals

CAUTIONS
• Shoulder issues

PERFECT YOUR FORM
• Avoid tensing your shoulders up to your ears.
• Avoid allowing your shoulder blades to lift off the floor. If your shoulder comes up, bend the arm of the lifted shoulder, and place your hand beneath your ribs for support.

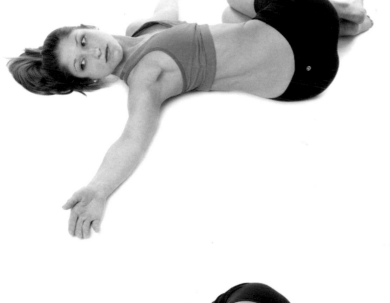

PARIVRTTA JANU SIRSASANA

INTERMEDIATE

(Revolved Head-to-Knee Pose)

PARIVRTTA JANU SIRSASANA, or Revolved Head-to-Knee Pose, is an intense seated side bend and twist that improves your flexibility. It stretches your obliques, shoulders, spine, and hamstrings and expands the intercostal muscles within your ribs, which can lead to greater lung capacity. Practicing this asana will leave you feeling limber and calm.

ANNOTATION KEY
Black text indicates strengthening muscles
Gray text indicates stretching muscles
----indicates deep muscles

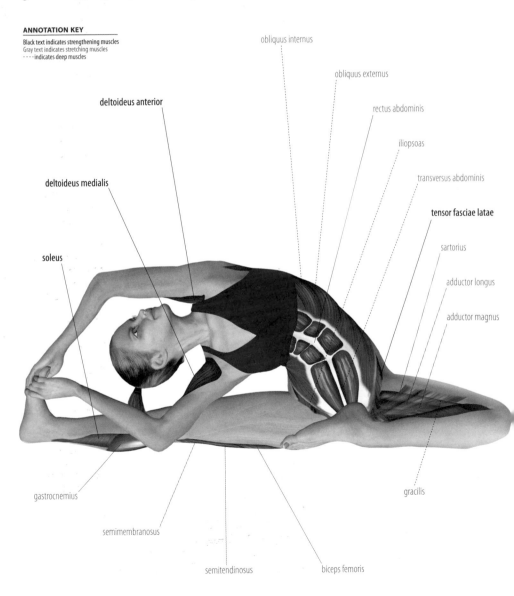

obliquus internus

obliquus externus

rectus abdominis

iliopsoas

deltoideus anterior

transversus abdominis

deltoideus medialis

tensor fasciae latae

sartorius

soleus

adductor longus

adductor magnus

gracilis

gastrocnemius

semimembranosus

semitendinosus

biceps femoris

HOW TO DO IT

1 Sit in Dandasana (see page 19), and then separate your legs as wide as you can. Bend your left knee, and draw your heel toward your groin, placing the sole of your foot on your right inner thigh. Lower your left knee to the floor. Draw both sit bones to the floor.

2 Inhale, and lift up through your spine. Exhale, and stretch toward your right leg. Flex your foot, and contract the muscles in your right thigh to push the back of your leg toward the floor. Make sure that your knee is pointed toward the ceiling.

3 Gently draw your right shoulder to your right inner thigh, and grasp the ball of your foot with your right hand. Keeping your right knee straight, lower your elbow to the floor. Rotate your torso toward the ceiling.

4 Inhale, and stretch your left arm up and over your head to grasp your right foot. Exhale, and press your left shoulder backward to rotate your torso further. Stretch deeper with each exhalation. Gaze toward the ceiling.

5 Hold for 30 seconds to 1 minute. Repeat with your left leg straight and your right leg bent.

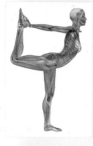

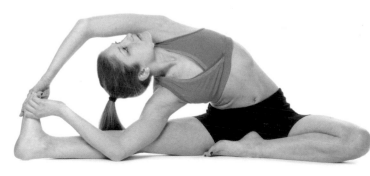

PRIMARY TARGETS
- gluteus medius
- obliquus internus
- adductor longus
- adductor magnus
- tibialis anterior
- gracilis
- rhomboideus
- trapezius
- latissimus dorsi
- erector spinae
- infraspinatus
- soleus
- gastrocnemius
- semimembranosus
- semitendinosus
- biceps femoris

BENEFITS
- Stretches hamstrings, groins, shoulders, and spine
- Stimulates digestion

CAUTIONS
- Knee injury
- Shoulder injury

PERFECT YOUR FORM
- Elongate the back of your neck.
- Open your chest to extend the arch through your entire spine.
- Avoid bending your extended knees.
- Don't hold your breath.

ARDHA MATSYENDRASANA

INTERMEDIATE

(Half Lord of the Fishes Pose; Spine-Twisting Pose)

ARDHA MATSYENDRASANA, most commonly known as Half Lord of the Fishes or Spine-Twisting Pose, offers a full-spine lateral twist. It is named for Matsyendra, a legendary teacher of yoga whose name translates to "king of the fish."

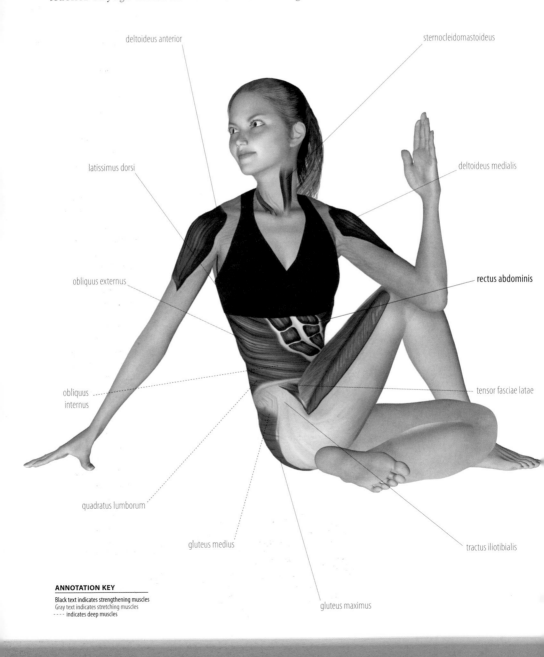

deltoideus anterior

sternocleidomastoideus

latissimus dorsi

deltoideus medialis

obliquus externus

rectus abdominis

obliquus internus

tensor fasciae latae

quadratus lumborum

tractus iliotibialis

gluteus medius

gluteus maximus

ANNOTATION KEY

Black text indicates strengthening muscles
Gray text indicates stretching muscles
- - - - indicates deep muscles

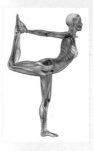

HOW TO DO IT

1 Sit in Dandasana (see page 19). Bend your right knee, and place your right foot over your left leg. Your right foot should be flat on the floor outside of your left thigh.

2 At the same time, bend your left knee, resting the outside of your left thigh on the floor. Your left heel should point toward your right sit bone.

3 Inhale, and lift up through your spine and chest while keeping your shoulders relaxed. Exhale, and begin twisting to your right. Place your left elbow on the outside of your right knee. Press your right hand on the floor behind your hips. Turn your head to the right.

4 Twist deeper with each exhalation. Lean back slightly, leading with your upper torso. Using your left arm, pull your right thigh closer toward your abdominals. Continue to lengthen your spine from the bottom up, pulling your

tailbone down. Use your right hand to guide your rotation deeper.

5 Hold for 30 seconds to 1 minute. Gently untwist as you exhale, and repeat with your left leg over your right thigh.

An easier variation of this pose is to keep your bottom leg straight. If you have trouble keeping both sit bones on the floor when drawing the heel of your bottom leg toward your sit bone, keep your leg extended out in front of you. Draw both sit bones to the floor and elongate your spine before twisting your torso.

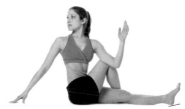

PRIMARY TARGETS
• rhomboideus
• sternocleidomastoideus
• latissimus dorsi
• erector spinae
• quadratus lumborum
• iliopsoas
• adductor longus
• obliquus internus
• obliquus externus

BENEFITS
• Stimulates digestion
• Stretches hips, spine, and shoulders
• Relieves backache and menstrual discomfort

CAUTIONS
• Back injury

PERFECT YOUR FORM
• Try to pull the thigh of your raised leg and your torso as close together as possible without collapsing your spine.
• Pull your back shoulder toward the back wall as you twist through your entire spine.
• Avoid rounding your spine.
• Avoid lifting the foot of your raised leg off the floor.

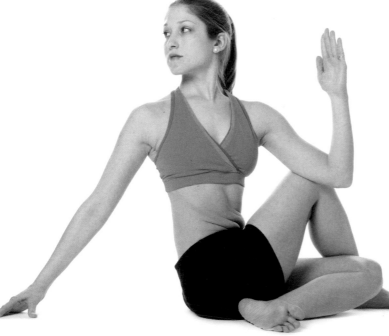

GOMUKHASANA

INTERMEDIATE

(Cow-Face Pose)

GOMUKHASANA, OR COW FACE POSE, is a seated posture that targets both your hips and shoulders. It is a multipurpose stretch that works the back of your arms, rotator cuff, upper back, glutes, hip rotators, and chest muscles. One explanation for this asana's name is that while in this posture, your thighs and calves resemble a cow's face.

ANNOTATION KEY
Black text indicates strengthening muscles
Gray text indicates stretching muscles
- - - - indicates deep muscles

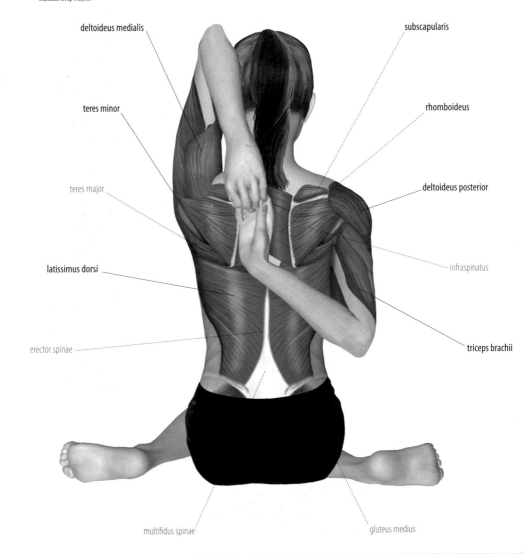

deltoideus medialis

subscapularis

teres minor

rhomboideus

teres major

deltoideus posterior

latissimus dorsi

infraspinatus

erector spinae

triceps brachii

multifidus spinae

gluteus medius

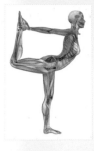

HOW TO DO IT

1 Sit in Agnistabbhasana (see page 20), with your right leg stacked on top of your left.

2 Slide your left ankle to the left and your right ankle to the right so that your knees are stacked on top of each other.

3 Lift up from your spine, sitting with equal weight on your sit bones. Inhale, and reach your right hand to the side, parallel to the floor.

4 Bend your elbow, and rotate your shoulder downward so that the palm of your hand faces behind you. Reach behind your back, palm still up, and draw your elbow into your right side. Continue to rotate your shoulder downward as you reach upward with your hand until your forearm is parallel to your spine. Your right hand should rest in between your shoulder blades.

5 With your next inhalation, reach your left arm up toward the ceiling with your palm facing outward. Exhale, and bend your elbow, reaching your left hand down the center of your back.

6 Hook your hands together behind your back. Lift your chest, and pull your abdominals in toward your spine.

7 Hold for approximately 1 minute. Repeat with your left leg stacked on top of your right, and your right elbow pointed toward the ceiling.

PRIMARY TARGETS
- deltoideus posterior
- deltoideus medialis
- teres minor
- rhomboideus
- subscapularis
- latissimus dorsi
- triceps brachii

BENEFITS
- Stretches hips, thighs, shoulders, and triceps

CAUTIONS
- Shoulder injury

PERFECT YOUR FORM
- Allow gravity to stretch your hips open.
- Make sure that whichever leg is on top, the opposite elbow is pointed toward the ceiling.
- If you cannot hook your hands behind your back, try using a strap to help you pull your hands closer together.
- Avoid lifting your sit bones off the floor.

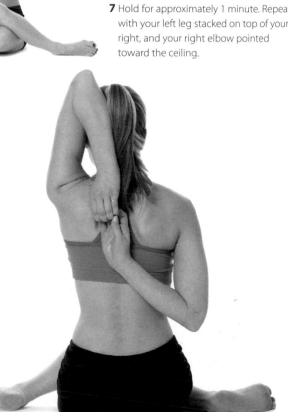

PARIPURNA NAVASANA

INTERMEDIATE

(Full Boat Pose)

PARIPURNA NAVASANA, or Full Boat Pose, is a confidence-boosting asana that challenges your core strength and demands both flexibility and endurance. It tones and strengthens your abdominal muscles, spine, and hip flexors while offering your hamstrings an efficient stretch.

ANNOTATION KEY

Black text indicates strengthening muscles
Gray text indicates stretching muscles
- - - - indicates deep muscles

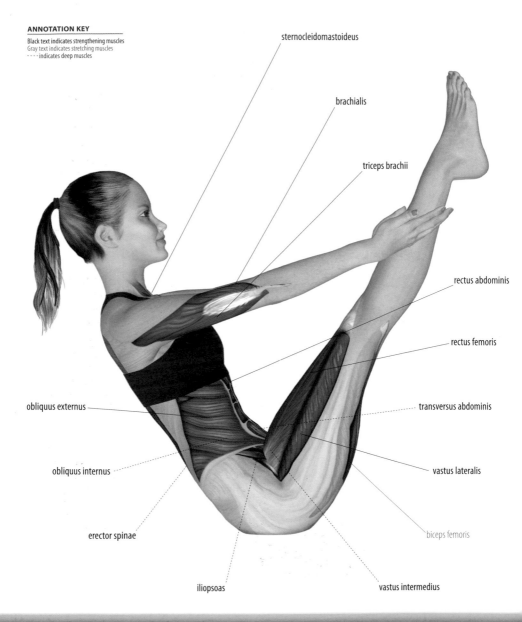

sternocleidomastoideus

brachialis

triceps brachii

rectus abdominis

rectus femoris

obliquus externus

transversus abdominis

obliquus internus

vastus lateralis

erector spinae

biceps femoris

iliopsoas

vastus intermedius

HOW TO DO IT

1 Sit in Dandasana (see page 19). Lean back slightly, bending your knees, and support yourself with your hands behind your hips. Your fingers should be pointing forward, and your back should be straight.

2 Exhale, and lift your feet off the floor as you lean back from your shoulders. Find your balance point between your sit bones and your tailbone.

3 Slowly straighten your legs in front of you so that they form a 45-degree angle with your torso. Point your toes. Lift your arms to your sides, parallel to the floor.

4 Pull your abdominals in toward your spine as they work to keep you balanced. With your palms facing up, stretch your arms forward through your fingertips, and elongate the back of your neck.

5 Hold for 10 to 20 seconds.

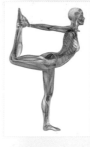

PRIMARY TARGETS
- rectus abdominis
- obliquus internus
- obliquus externus
- iliopsoas
- transversus abdominis
- vastus intermedius
- rectus femoris
- erector spinae

BENEFITS
- Strengthens abdominals, hip flexors, spine, and thighs
- Stretches hamstrings
- Stimulates digestion
- Alleviates thyroid problems

CAUTIONS
- Neck injury
- Headache
- Lower back pain

PERFECT YOUR FORM
- Keep your neck elongated and relaxed, minimizing the tension in your upper spine.
- If you are unable to straighten your legs, balance with your knees bent.
- Avoid rounding your spine, causing you to sink into your lower back.

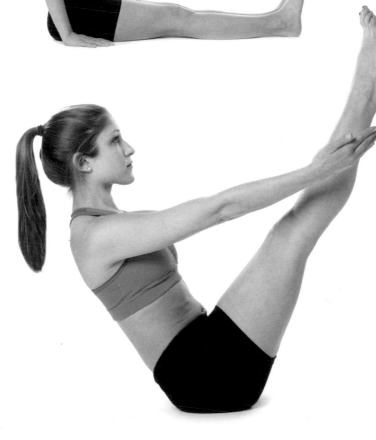

PADMASANA

ADVANCED

(Lotus Pose)

THE YOGA CLASSIC, PADMASANA, or Lotus Pose, is the ultimate meditation pose. Padmasana allows you to hold your body steady for long periods, allowing you to calm your mind. As well as facilitating meditation, this cross-legged sitting asana opens up your hips and stretches your ankles and knees. It looks simple, but beginners may find it difficult, so go at your own pace, honing your skills of concentration and focus.

ANNOTATION KEY

Black text indicates strengthening muscles
Gray text indicates stretching muscles
- - - - indicates deep muscles

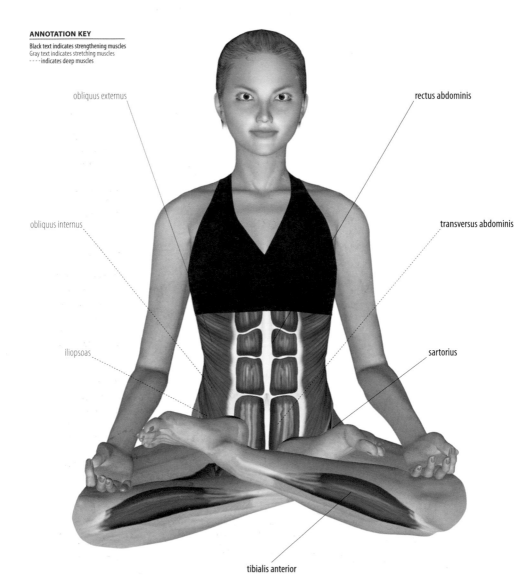

obliquus externus

rectus abdominis

obliquus internus

transversus abdominis

iliopsoas

sartorius

tibialis anterior

HOW TO DO IT

1 Sit in Dandasana (see page 19). Lift up through your spine.

2 Bend your right knee and open it to the side. Allow your hip to open, and lower your right thigh to the floor.

3 Lean forward slightly, and grab your right shin with your hands. Place your right foot on top of your left thigh, with your heel nestled against your groin. Make sure that the rotation is coming from your hips.

4 Carefully position your left foot beneath your right thigh. Draw your knees closer together. Push into the floor with your groins, as you keep both sit bones on the floor. This is Ardha Padmasana, or the Half Lotus Pose.

5 To continue to Padmasana, the full expression of the Lotus Pose, extend your left leg from below your right hip. With your knee bent, grab your left shin with your hands. Lean back slightly as you bring your left shin on top of your right, and place your left foot on top of your right thigh. Nestle your left heel against your right groin.

6 Push into the floor with your groins and rotate your hips open to press your thighs to the floor. Be sure to keep both sit bones on the floor.

7 Extend upward through your spine and place the backs of your hands on each knee, forming an "O" with each index finger and thumb.

8 Hold for 5 seconds to 1 minute. Repeat with your right leg on top.

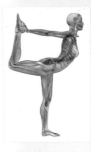

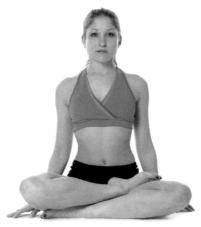

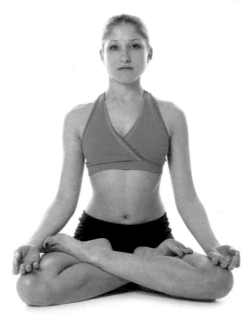

PRIMARY TARGETS
- rectus abdominis
- transversus abdominis
- tibialis anterior
- sartorius
- rectus femoris

BENEFITS
- Stretches hips, thighs, knees, and ankles
- Stimulates digestion
- Calms the brain for meditation

CAUTIONS
- Knee injury
- Hip injury
- Ankle injury

PERFECT YOUR FORM
- Hold the position for the same length of time on both sides.
- If you experience hip or knee discomfort in this position, practice Ardha Padmasana (see step 4) or Baddha Konasana (see pages 68–69) until your hips and knees are flexible enough to come into full Padmasana.
- If you have trouble keeping your spine in a straight, neutral position, place a folded blanked beneath your hips to elevate your hips above your knees.

HANUMANASANA

ADVANCED   *(Monkey Pose; Front Splits Pose)*

HANUMANASANA, OR MONKEY POSE, is also known as the Front Splits Pose. It stretches the hamstrings, groins, and hip flexors and strengthens the pelvic floor muscles and abdominals. Hanumanasana is a true yoga challenge, so go slowly as you learn this pose—it may take months or even years for you to master it.

ANNOTATION KEY

Black text indicates strengthening muscles
Gray text indicates stretching muscles
- - - -indicates deep muscles

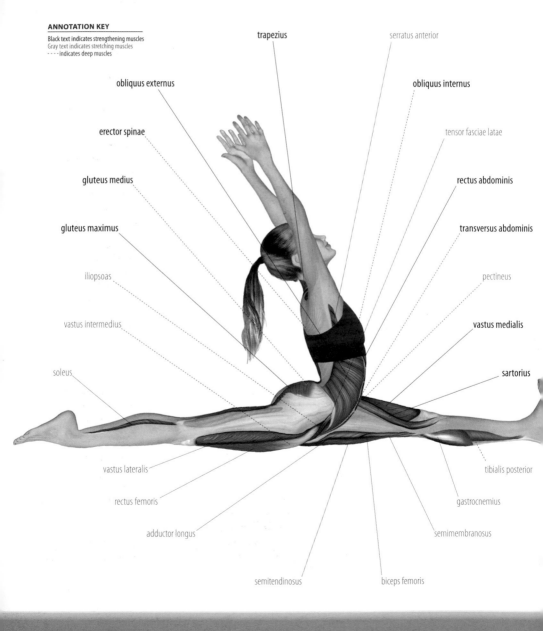

trapezius

serratus anterior

obliquus externus

obliquus internus

erector spinae

tensor fasciae latae

gluteus medius

rectus abdominis

gluteus maximus

transversus abdominis

iliopsoas

pectineus

vastus intermedius

vastus medialis

soleus

sartorius

vastus lateralis

tibialis posterior

rectus femoris

gastrocnemius

adductor longus

semimembranosus

semitendinosus

biceps femoris

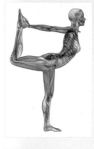

HOW TO DO IT

1 Kneel on the floor with your hips open and your back straight.

2 Place your left foot on the floor in front of you to create a lunge position. Make sure that your hips are aligned and facing forward.

3 Lean forward slightly to balance on your fingertips. Slowly extend your right leg behind you while simultaneously extending your left leg forward.

4 When you have fully lowered yourself to the floor, straighten both legs completely, and point your toes. Your right knee should be facing the floor, and your left knee should face the ceiling. Your hips should be parallel and facing forward.

5 Lift your chest, and raise your arms toward the ceiling. Arch your back slightly with your shoulders open.

6 Hold for 30 seconds to 1 minute. Repeat with your right leg in front.

PRIMARY TARGETS
- iliopsoas
- pectineus
- adductor longus
- sartorius
- vastus intermedius
- rectus femoris
- biceps femoris
- semimembranosus
- semitendinosus

BENEFITS
- Stretches hamstrings and groins

CAUTIONS
- Groin injury
- Hamstring injury

PERFECT YOUR FORM
- Practice on a hardwood floor or another smooth surface so that you can slide more easily into the pose.
- Push into the floor with your front heel and the top of your back foot as you descend.
- Avoid pushing yourself too far into the pose—only stretch as far as your hamstrings allow.
- Avoid turning your hips out to the side.

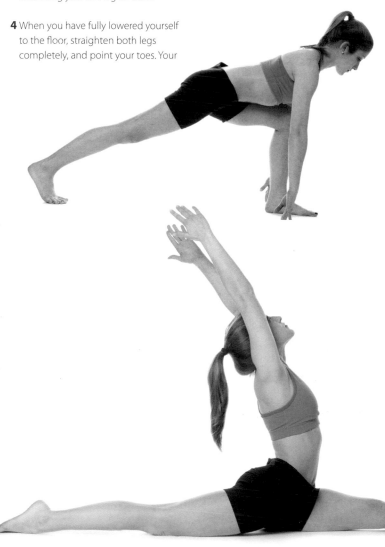

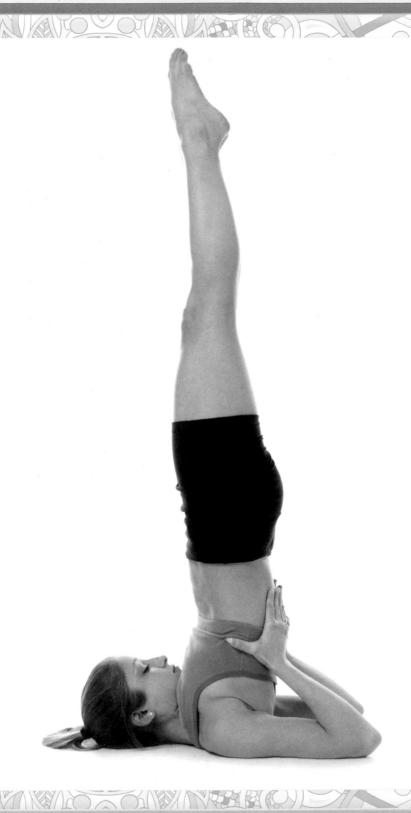

ARM SUPPORTS & INVERSIONS

As you age, your bones and upper-body strength deteriorate, increasing your risk of injury and making everyday tasks more difficult. Arm supports work to reverse the weakening of bones and muscles. These poses strengthen your arms, shoulders, and chest, and they help prevent osteoporosis. You will also strengthen your abdominals as you engage them to balance and support your body. Arm supports do require a degree of flexibility, especially in your spine and hips. Let go of any unnecessary tension—the fear of falling on your face is natural. Overcome the fear by building your upper-body strength with diligent practice.

Inversions move your head below your heart, reversing the effects of gravity on your body. Inversions benefit the cardiovascular, lymphatic, nervous, and endocrine systems, increasing blood circulation and building healthier lung tissue. When beginning inversions, start by holding them for short periods, adding more time as your body adapts. And always be gentle on your neck.

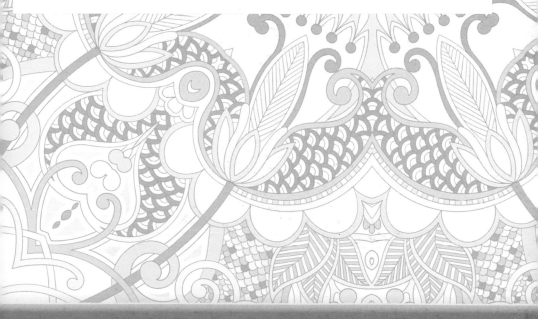

PLANK POSE TO CHATURANGA DANDASANA

(Plank Pose to Four-Limbed Staff Pose)

PLANK POSE is one of the foundation asanas of yoga, teaching you to hold your body steady and firm—like a strong wooden plank. You can practice it on its own, but it is also part of the Sun Salutations, followed by Chaturanga Dandasana, or Four-Limbed Staff Pose, another essential foundation asana. Chaturanga is the yoga version of a push-up. Both Plank Pose and Chaturanga strengthen your abdominals, as well as your arms and wrists, preparing you for more advanced arm supports.

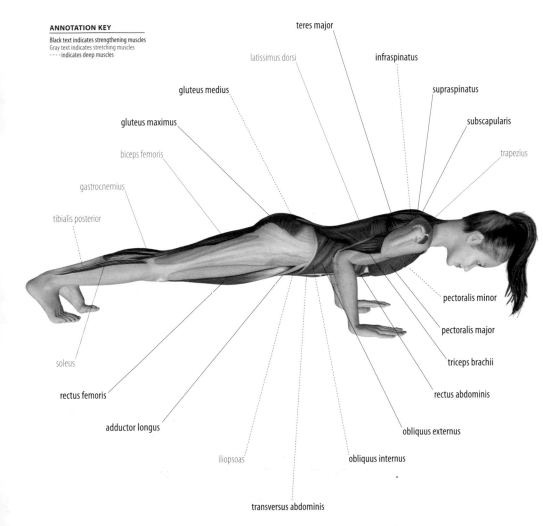

ANNOTATION KEY
Black text indicates strengthening muscles
Gray text indicates stretching muscles
----indicates deep muscles

teres major

latissimus dorsi

infraspinatus

supraspinatus

gluteus medius

subscapularis

gluteus maximus

trapezius

biceps femoris

gastrocnemius

tibialis posterior

pectoralis minor

pectoralis major

triceps brachii

soleus

rectus abdominis

rectus femoris

adductor longus

obliquus externus

iliopsoas

obliquus internus

transversus abdominis

HOW TO DO IT

1 To assume Plank Pose, begin in Adho Mukha Svanasana (see page 22).

2 Inhale, and draw your torso forward until your wrists are directly under your shoulders at a 90-degree angle. Your body should form a straight line from the top of your head to your heels.

3 Press your hands firmly down into the floor, and, without letting your chest sink, press back through your heels.

4 Keeping your neck in line with your spine, broaden your shoulder blades. Your legs should be strong, straight, and engaged, and your feet should be square, with your heels pointing upward. Hold Plank Pose for 30 seconds to 1 minute.

5 To move into Chaturanga, open your chest, and broaden your shoulder blades while tucking in your tailbone.

6 Exhale, and with your legs turned slightly inward, lower yourself toward the floor until your upper arms are parallel to your spine.

7 Tuck your tailbone under, and draw your abdominals in toward your spine to maintain the straight line from your shoulders to your heels. Keep your elbows in by your sides. Lift your head and look forward.

8 Hold for 10 to 30 seconds.

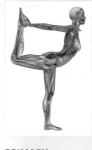

PRIMARY TARGETS
- rectus abdominis
- triceps brachii
- subscapularis
- supraspinatus
- infraspinatus
- teres major
- pectoralis major
- pectoralis minor

BENEFITS
- Strengthens and tones arms and abdominals
- Strengthens wrists

CAUTIONS
- Shoulder issues
- Wrist injury
- Lower-back injury

PERFECT YOUR FORM
- Lengthen your legs all the way through your heels to evenly distribute weight while in Plank Pose.
- Squeeze your glutes, and draw in your abdominals for stability.
- Avoid sinking your shoulders.
- Avoid sagging your hips or raising your buttocks.
- Avoid hunching your shoulders up toward your ears.

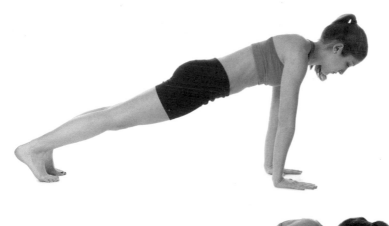

VASISTHASANA

INTERMEDIATE *(Side Plank Pose; Sage Pose; One-Arm Balance; Inclined Plank)*

NAMED FOR VASISTH, a venerated sage, Vasisthasana is a powerful asana that strengthens your arms and enhances your balance. In its fullest version, your top leg is raised perpendicular to the floor—a posture only for the most advanced yoga practitioner. Also known as Side Plank, Inclined Plank, and One-Arm Balance, this asana will leave you feeling rejuvenated in body, mind, and spirit.

ANNOTATION KEY
Black text indicates strengthening muscles
Gray text indicates stretching muscles
- - - - indicates deep muscles

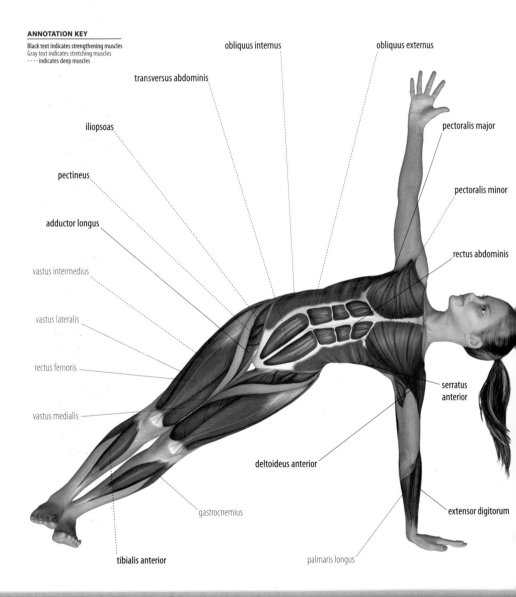

obliquus internus

obliquus externus

transversus abdominis

iliopsoas

pectineus

adductor longus

vastus intermedius

vastus lateralis

rectus femoris

vastus medialis

pectoralis major

pectoralis minor

rectus abdominis

serratus anterior

deltoideus anterior

gastrocnemius

tibialis anterior

palmaris longus

extensor digitorum

HOW TO DO IT

1 Begin in Plank Pose (see pages 128–129). Your arms should be straight, with your wrists aligned under your shoulders. To prepare for Vasisthasana, you may want your hands slightly in front of your shoulders to push into for support.

2 Shift your weight onto the outside of your right foot and onto your right arm. Roll to the side, guiding with your hips and bringing your left shoulder back. Stack your left foot on top of the right, squeezing both legs together and straight.

3 Exhale, bring your left arm up toward the ceiling, and elongate your body, making a straight line from your head to your heels. Gaze up at your fingertips as you continue to push through your shoulder into the floor, maintaining a strong balance.

4 Breathe, and hold the posture for 15 to 30 seconds. Return to Plank Pose or Adho Mukha Svanasana (see page 22), and repeat on the left side.

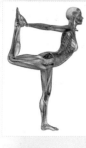

PRIMARY TARGETS

- rectus abdominis
- obliquus internus
- obliquus externus
- transversus abdominis
- pectoralis major
- pectoralis minor
- serratus anterior
- deltoideus anterior
- extensor digitorum

BENEFITS

- Strengthens wrists, arms, legs, and abdominals
- Improves balance

CAUTIONS

- Shoulder issues
- Wrist injury
- Elbow injury

PERFECT YOUR FORM

- Elongate your limbs as much as possible, stretching through your legs into the floor and reaching your top arm high to the ceiling.
- Your feet should be stacked and flexed as if they were side by side in standing position.
- Avoid allowing your hips or shoulders to sway or sink.
- Avoid lifting your hips too high.

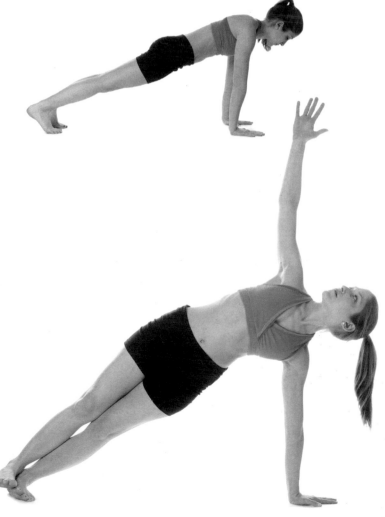

PURVOTTANASANA

INTERMEDIATE

(Upward Plank Pose; Eastern Stretch)

PURVOTTANASANA, OR UPWARD PLANK POSE, is an effective heart opener that stretches your chest and shoulders and strengthens your legs and arms. It works as a counterpose to Chaturanga by stretching your pectoralis major, pectoralis minor, and deltoideus anterior, which tightly contract in the push-up position. It also works well as a follow-up to forward-bending postures.

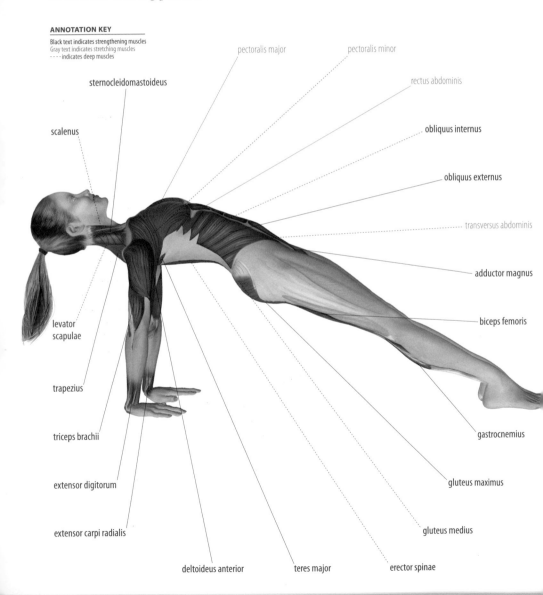

ANNOTATION KEY

Black text indicates strengthening muscles
Gray text indicates stretching muscles
- - - - indicates deep muscles

pectoralis major

pectoralis minor

rectus abdominis

sternocleidomastoideus

obliquus internus

scalenus

obliquus externus

transversus abdominis

adductor magnus

biceps femoris

levator scapulae

trapezius

gastrocnemius

triceps brachii

gluteus maximus

extensor digitorum

gluteus medius

extensor carpi radialis

deltoideus anterior

teres major

erector spinae

HOW TO DO IT

1 Sitting in Dandasana (see page 19) with your legs extended, place the palms of your hands on the floor several inches behind your hips, fingers facing forward.

2 Draw your knees toward your chest, and place your feet on the floor with your heels about a foot away from your buttocks, and turn your big toes slightly inward.

3 Exhale, pressing down with your hands and feet and lifting your hips until your back and thighs are parallel to the floor. Your shoulders should be directly above your wrists.

4 Without lowering your hips, straighten your legs one at a time.

5 Lifting your chest and bringing your shoulder blades together, push your hips higher, creating a slight arch in your back. Do not squeeze your buttocks to create the lift.

6 Slowly and gently elongate your neck and let it drop back.

7 Hold for 30 seconds to 1 minute and return to Dandasana.

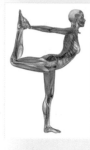

PRIMARY TARGETS
• deltoideus anterior
• triceps brachii
• teres major
• teres minor
• erector spinae
• gluteus maximus
• gluteus medius
• adductor magnus
• biceps femoris
• pectoralis minor

BENEFITS
• Strengthens the spine, arms, and hamstrings
• Extends the hips and chest

CAUTIONS
• Neck injury
• Wrist injury

PERFECT YOUR FORM
• Avoid using your glutes to maintain the position.
• Avoid sagging your hips.

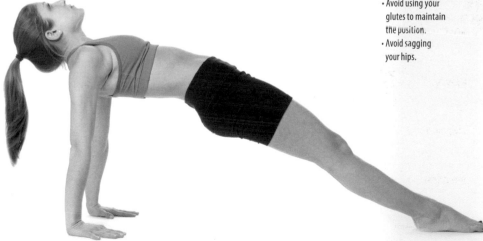

HALASANA

BEGINNER

(Plow Pose)

HALASANA, OR PLOW POSE, is a great introduction to yoga inversions. It primarily works to enhance spinal flexibility, but if you are a beginner, it may take time and practice for you to lift your legs to touch the floor behind your head. Go slowly to avoid strain on your cervical spine. When done properly, Halasana also increases circulation and vitality, while strengthening the abdomen and preparing you for relaxation and meditation.

ANNOTATION KEY

Black text indicates strengthening muscles
Gray text indicates stretching muscles
----indicates deep muscles

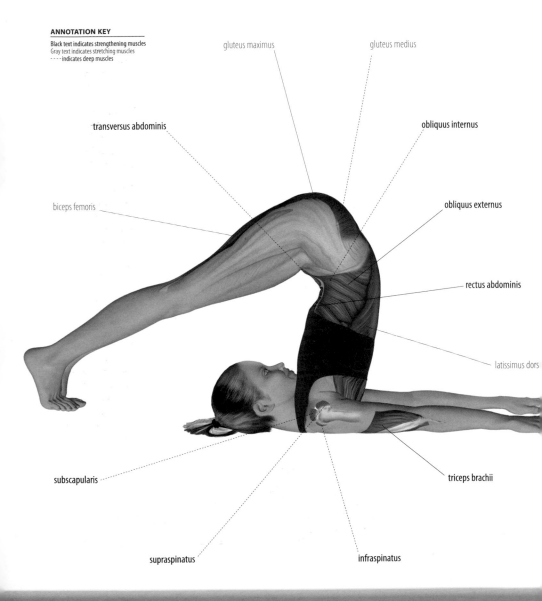

gluteus maximus

gluteus medius

transversus abdominis

obliquus internus

biceps femoris

obliquus externus

rectus abdominis

latissimus dorsi

subscapularis

triceps brachii

supraspinatus

infraspinatus

HOW TO DO IT

1 Lie supine on the floor with your knees bent. Your arms should be by your sides, with your hands placed flat on the floor.

2 Tighten your abdominals, and lift your knees off the floor. Exhale, press your arms into the floor, and lift your knees higher so that your buttocks and hips come off the floor.

3 Continue lifting your knees toward your face, and roll your back off the mat from your hips to your shoulders. With your upper arms firmly planted on the floor, bend your elbows, and place your hands on your lower back. Draw your elbows in closer to your sides.

4 Inhale, tuck your tailbone toward your pubis, and straighten your legs back toward your head. Your torso should be perpendicular to the floor.

5 Exhale, and continue to extend your legs beyond your head. Squeeze your legs and bend at your waist until your toes touch the floor. Place your hands face down on the floor, pushing through your arms to maintain the lift in your hips.

6 Hold for 1 to 5 minutes.

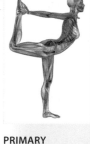

PRIMARY TARGETS
• rectus abdominis
• latissimus dorsi
• transversus abdominis
• triceps brachii
• infraspinatus
• supraspinatus
• subscapularis

BENEFITS
• Relieves stress
• Relieves backache and headache
• Stimulates digestion

CAUTIONS
• High blood pressure
• Neck issues
• Menstruation or pregnancy

PERFECT YOUR FORM
• Soften your throat, and relax your tongue.
• If your toes don't reach the floor, continue supporting your back with your hands.
• Place folded blankets below your shoulders if the posture strains your neck.
• Avoid swinging your legs down quickly into the pose.

SALAMBA SARVANGASANA

INTERMEDIATE

(Supported Shoulderstand)

IF YOUR BACK AND SHOULDERS are tight, Salamba Sarvangasana, or Supported Shoulderstand, will be a challenge, but mastering this pose yields many benefits. Yoga inversions improve your balance, concentration, and circulation, and also calm and hydrate the body.

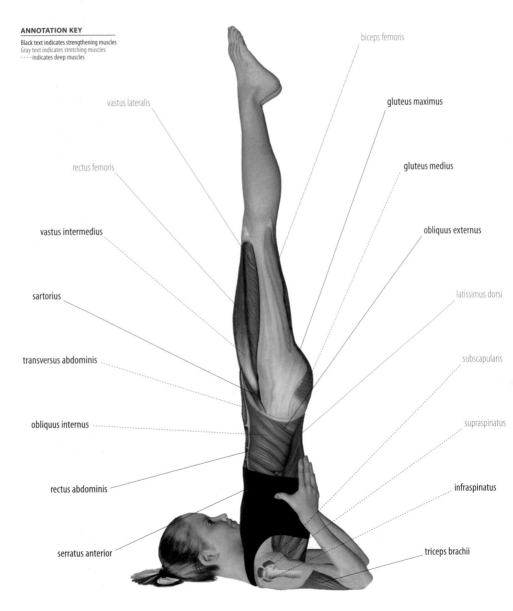

ANNOTATION KEY
Black text indicates strengthening muscles
Gray text indicates stretching muscles
----indicates deep muscles

biceps femoris

vastus lateralis

gluteus maximus

rectus femoris

gluteus medius

vastus intermedius

obliquus externus

sartorius

latissimus dorsi

transversus abdominis

subscapularis

obliquus internus

supraspinatus

rectus abdominis

infraspinatus

serratus anterior

triceps brachii

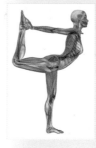

HOW TO DO IT

1 Lie supine on the floor with your knees bent and arms by your sides.

2 Tighten your abdominals, and lift your knees off the floor. Exhale, press your arms into the floor, and lift your knees higher so that your buttocks come off the floor.

3 Continue lifting your knees toward your face, and roll your back off the mat from your hips to your shoulders. With your upper arms firmly planted on the floor, bend your elbows, and place your hands on your lower back. Draw your elbows in closer to your sides.

4 Inhale, tuck your tailbone toward your pubis, and straighten your legs back toward your head. Your torso should be perpendicular to the floor.

5 With your next inhalation, extend your legs up toward the ceiling, opening your hips as you lift. Squeeze your buttocks, and press down with your elbows to create a straight, elongated line from your chest to your toes.

6 Hold for 30 seconds to 5 minutes before bending your knees and hips and returning to the floor.

PRIMARY TARGETS
• rectus abdominis
• transversus abdominis
• biceps femoris
• sartorius
• supraspinatus
• infraspinatus
• subscapularis
• triceps brachii
• latissimus dorsi
• gluteus maximus
• gluteus medius

BENEFITS
• Relieves stress
• Stretches shoulders and cervical spine
• Stimulates digestion
• Relieves symptoms of menopause

CAUTIONS
• High blood pressure
• Neck issues
• Headache or ear infection

PERFECT YOUR FORM
• Soften your throat, and relax your tongue.
• If you can't lift your pelvis into the inversion, practice a few feet away from a wall and walk your feet up the wall until you can place your hands on your back.
• Place folded blankets below your shoulders if the posture strains your neck.

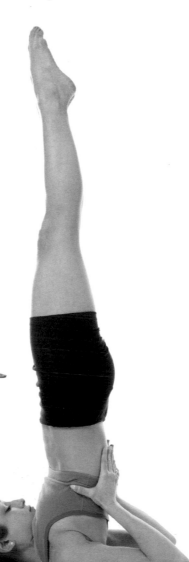

SALAMBA SIRSASANA

INTERMEDIATE

(Supported Headstand)

YOGA INVERSIONS, such as Salamba Sirsasana, or the Supported Headstand, can be intimidating—they ask you to literally look at the world upside-down. But overcoming the fear of the unfamiliar is part of yoga. Practicing Tadasana (see pages 30–31) is actually the best preparation for this gravity-reversing asana—you'll need the same strong alignment of the legs, torso, and neck.

ANNOTATION KEY
Black text indicates strengthening muscles
Gray text indicates stretching muscles
----indicates deep muscles

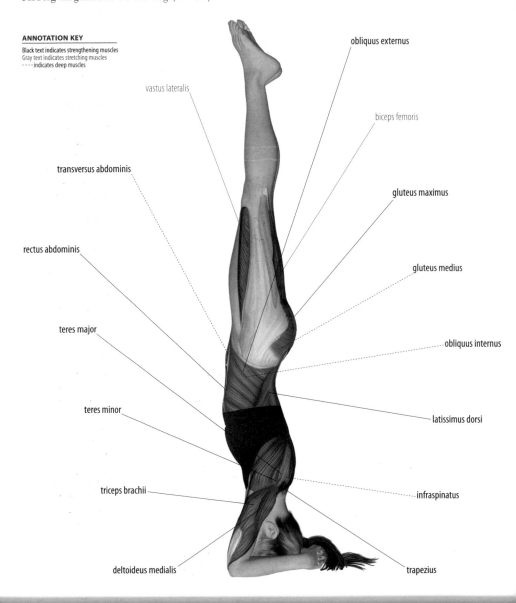

obliquus externus

vastus lateralis

biceps femoris

transversus abdominis

gluteus maximus

rectus abdominis

gluteus medius

teres major

obliquus internus

teres minor

latissimus dorsi

triceps brachii

infraspinatus

deltoideus medialis

trapezius

HOW TO DO IT

1 Kneel on the floor. Your hips should be lifted off your heels.

2 Place your hands on the floor in front of you and lower your elbows to the floor, keeping them in by your sides and aligned with your shoulders.

3 Exhale, and lift your knees off the floor. Ground your feet flat on the floor, pushing your heels down.

4 Straighten your legs as you lift your sit bones to the ceiling. Tuck your tailbone toward your pubis, and squeeze your legs together.

5 Inhale, and slowly walk toward your head on the balls of your feet, causing your hips to lift toward the ceiling.

6 Once your weight has shifted to your shoulders and forearms, lift your feet off the floor. Use your abdominals to slowly raise both legs simultaneously.

7 Lengthening your spine and keeping your shoulders open, bend your knees and draw your thighs toward your abdominals. Take a few calming breaths, and balance in this position.

8 Exhale, and slowly lift your toes toward the ceiling. Tuck your tailbone toward your pubis while pulling your abdominals in toward your spine. Elongate your entire body from the top of your neck through your toes.

9 Hold for 10 seconds to 3 minutes. To come out of the pose, exhale, and lower your feet to the floor simultaneously.

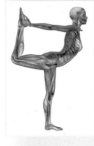

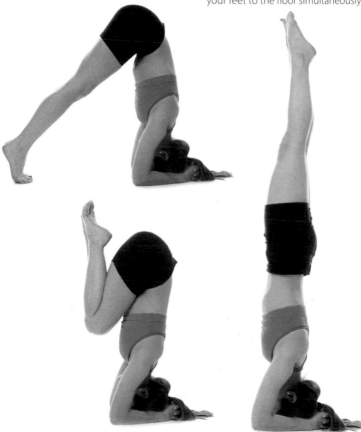

PRIMARY TARGETS
- rectus abdominis
- transversus abdominis
- latissimus dorsi
- gluteus medius
- trapezius
- deltoideus medialis
- infraspinatus
- triceps brachii

BENEFITS
- Strengthens and tones abdominals
- Strengthens arms, legs, and spine
- Improves balance

CAUTIONS
- Back injury
- Neck injury
- Headache
- High blood pressure

PERFECT YOUR FORM
- Support your weight evenly between your forearms.
- Be careful to not put too much weight on your neck or head.
- Don't jump into the pose or kick up to the headstand one foot at a time.
- If you have trouble balancing in the headstand, practice with the backs of your shoulders against a wall.

ARM SUPPORTS & INVERSIONS

BAKASANA

INTERMEDIATE

(Crow Pose; Crane Pose)

BAKASANA, KNOWN AS CROW POSE or Crane Pose, is an arm balance that challenges both your arm and core muscles. It looks harder than it is, but with concentration, you'll master this fun asana. For beginners, though, it is best to have a yoga instructor or another person at your side—because until you have upper-arm and abdominal strength, as well as fine balance, it is easy to tip over.

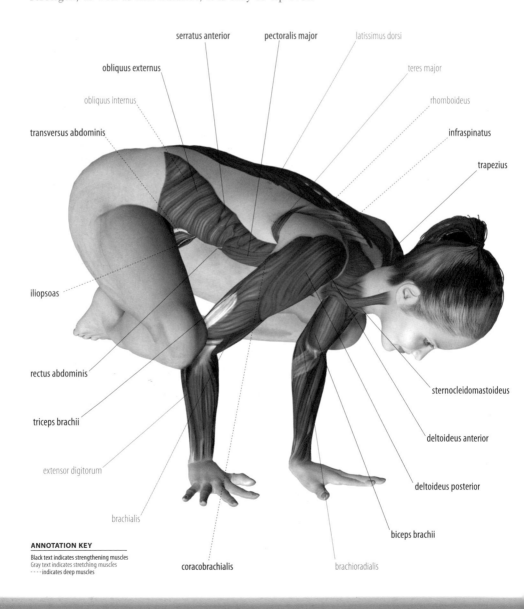

serratus anterior

pectoralis major

latissimus dorsi

obliquus externus

teres major

obliquus internus

rhomboideus

transversus abdominis

infraspinatus

trapezius

iliopsoas

rectus abdominis

sternocleidomastoideus

triceps brachii

deltoideus anterior

extensor digitorum

deltoideus posterior

brachialis

biceps brachii

ANNOTATION KEY
Black text indicates strengthening muscles
Gray text indicates stretching muscles
----indicates deep muscles

coracobrachialis

brachioradialis

HOW TO DO IT

1 Begin in Malasana (see pages 38–39), squatting with your feet and knees separated wider than your hips.

2 Lean your torso forward, and extend your arms to place your hands on the floor in front of you. Turn your hands inward slightly, and widen your fingers.

3 Bend your elbows, resting your knees against your upper arms. Lifting up on the balls of your feet and leaning your torso forward, bring your thighs toward your chest and your shins to your upper arms. Round your back as you feel your weight transfer to your wrists.

4 Exhale, and slowly lift your feet one at a time. Keep your head position neutral, and find your balance point.

5 Hold for 20 seconds to 1 minute.

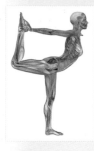

PRIMARY TARGETS
- iliopsoas
- trapezius
- serratus anterior
- deltoideus anterior
- deltoideus posterior
- triceps brachii
- biceps brachii
- coracobrachialis
- pectoralis major

BENEFITS
- Strengthens and tones arms and abdominals
- Strengthens wrists
- Improves balance

CAUTIONS
- Carpal tunnel syndrome
- Pregnancy

PERFECT YOUR FORM
- If you are afraid of falling forward, place a blanket in front of you as a cushion.
- Gaze at a spot on the floor in front of you to maintain balance.
- Avoid dropping your head.
- Don't jump into the posture.

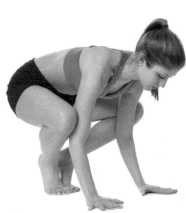

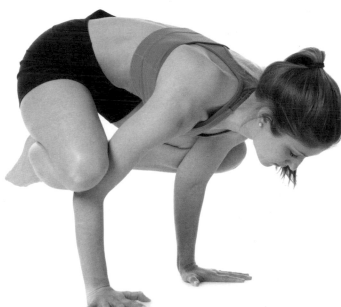

PARSVA BAKASANA

ADVANCED

(Side Crow Pose; Side Crane Pose)

PARSVA BAKASANA, known as the Side Crane Pose or Side Crow Pose, takes the balancing skills you've acquired in Bakasana a step further. This intense arm balance includes a deep twist, which will engage your obliques and abdominals, as well as your wrist, arm, shoulder, and chest muscles.

ANNOTATION KEY

Black text indicates strengthening muscles
Gray text indicates stretching muscles
- - - - indicates deep muscles

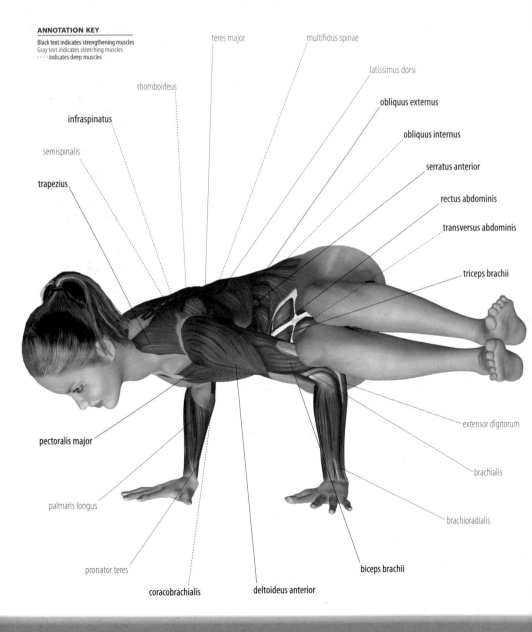

teres major

multifidus spinae

latissimus dorsi

obliquus externus

rhomboideus

obliquus internus

infraspinatus

serratus anterior

semispinalis

rectus abdominis

trapezius

transversus abdominis

triceps brachii

extensor digitorum

pectoralis major

brachialis

palmaris longus

brachioradialis

pronator teres

biceps brachii

coracobrachialis

deltoideus anterior

HOW TO DO IT

1 Stand in Samasthiti (see page 31), with your hands together at the middle of your chest. With your legs together, begin by squatting deeply until your buttocks are just above your heels, which are lifted off the floor.

2 Bring your arms across your body to your right side, touching your left elbow to your right thigh as your hands reach the floor. Exhale, and deepen the twist, pulling your right shoulder back.

4 Place your left hand flat on the floor outside your right thigh. Place the outside of your right thigh on your left upper arm. Lean to the right until you can place your right hand flat on the floor so that your hands are shoulder-width apart. Your hips and shoulders should maintain a deep twist.

5 Slowly lift your pelvis as you shift your weight toward your hands, using your left arm as a support for your right thigh. Continue shifting to the right, drawing your abdominals in toward your spine. Keep your feet together as you raise them completely off the floor toward your buttocks, exhaling.

6 Hold for 20 seconds to 1 minute, breathing through the balance. Exhale as you bring your feet to the floor. Repeat on the other side.

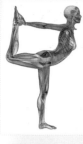

ARM SUPPORTS & INVERSIONS

PRIMARY TARGETS
- iliopsoas
- trapezius
- serratus anterior
- deltoideus anterior
- triceps brachii
- biceps brachii
- coracobrachialis
- pectoralis major
- obliquus internus

BENEFITS
- Strengthens and tones arms and abdominals
- Strengthens wrists
- Improves balance

CAUTIONS
- Wrist injury
- Lower-back injury

PERFECT YOUR FORM
- Gaze at a spot on the floor in front of you to maintain balance.
- Avoid dropping your head.
- Don't jump into the posture.

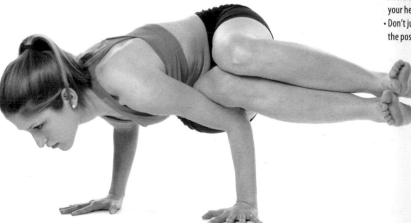

ASTAVAKRASANA

ADVANCED

(Eight-Angle Pose)

LIKE OTHER YOGA ARM BALANCES, Astavakrasana, or Eight-Angle Pose, will strengthen your wrists, arms, and core. One of the most advanced of the arm balances, Astavakrasana requires a great deal of stability and balance. Although it may take time to master, persevere and have fun working on the pose—another benefit of practice is the development of patience and fortitude.

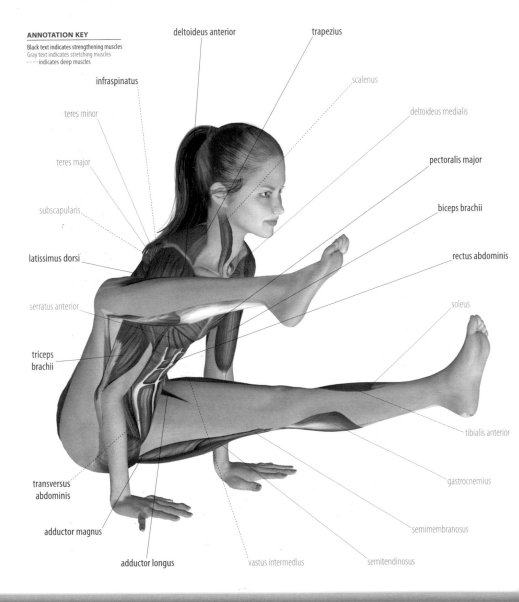

ANNOTATION KEY
Black text indicates strengthening muscles
Gray text indicates stretching muscles
- - - - indicates deep muscles

deltoideus anterior

trapezius

scalenus

infraspinatus

deltoideus medialis

teres minor

teres major

pectoralis major

subscapularis

biceps brachii

latissimus dorsi

rectus abdominis

serratus anterior

soleus

triceps
brachii

transversus
abdominis

tibialis anterior

gastrocnemius

adductor magnus

semimembranosus

adductor longus

vastus intermedius

semitendinosus

HOW TO DO IT

1 Sitting on the floor, open your hips, allowing your knees to lower toward the floor.

2 Lift your right leg, and bend it so that your thigh is perpendicular to the floor. Use your arms to pull your right leg over your right shoulder so that the back of your knee rests on top of your shoulder.

3 Lean your torso forward, and place your hands shoulder-width apart on the floor in front of you. Your right hand should be on the outside of your right leg.

4 Shift your weight forward onto your hands, and press up, lifting your chest through the movement. Straighten your left leg in front of you.

5 Exhale, and lower your torso until it is parallel to the floor. Draw your left leg toward the right. Bending both legs so that they lock at the ankles, hook your right ankle below the left.

6 Bend your arms and lower your chest toward the floor, squeezing your legs together and extending them to the right. Your thighs should be parallel to the floor, squeezing your right arm.

7 Twist your torso to the left, and keep your elbows in by your sides. Gaze at the floor in front of you.

8 Hold for 30 seconds to 1 minute. Slowly straighten your arms and lift your torso. Bend your knees, unhook your ankles, and return to a seated position on the floor. Repeat on the other side.

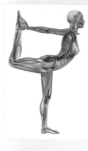

PRIMARY TARGETS
- adductor magnus
- adductor longus
- triceps brachii
- biceps brachii

BENEFITS
- Strengthens wrists, arms, and abdominals
- Increases balance and flexibility

CAUTIONS
- Shoulder issues
- Wrist injury
- Elbow injury

PERFECT YOUR FORM
- To keep your legs symmetrical, twist more from the spine than from your hips.
- If you struggle with keeping your body lifted off the floor, use blocks for your hands to practice pressing your hips up as one leg rests on your shoulder.
- Avoid allowing your top hip to rock backward, causing your bottom hip to drop.

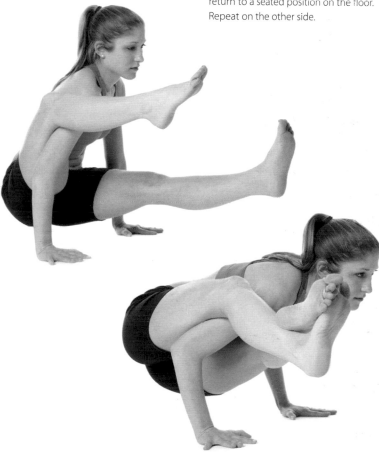

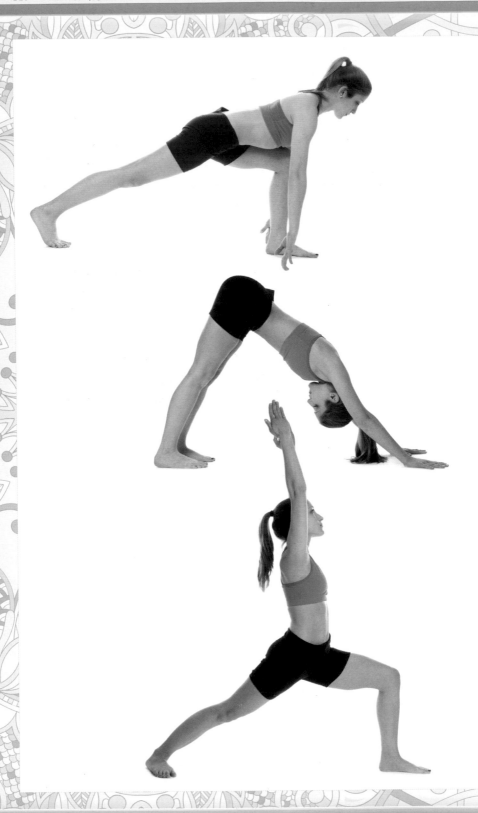

YOGA FLOWS

Familiarizing yourself with various yoga asanas is only the first step in your yoga practice. Incorporating these asanas into sequences, flowing from one pose to the next, allows you to maximize the strength and flexibility that you will gain throughout your entire body. Generally, yoga flows begin with gentler poses, build up to those that are more challenging, and end with a cooldown.

The traditional way to start your day is with an invigorating Surya Namasjara—better known as a Sun Salutation. For other yoga practice there are endless combinations of asanas, from those that calm your spirit to those that strengthen your body. The yoga flows shown in the following pages are just guides to get you started. With each individual asana, focus on attaining the proper body position before moving on. Combine other poses to add variety and create a yoga practice that best suits your body's needs.

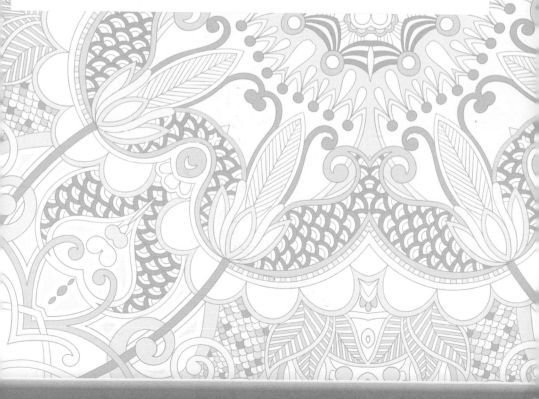

SURYA NAMASKARA A

This version of the classic Salute to the Sun makes
a perfect wake-up flow for practitioners of all levels.

(Sun Salutation A)

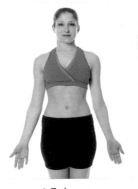

1 Tadasana

page 30

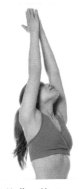

2 Urdhva Hastasana

page 24

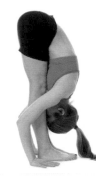

3 Uttanasana

page 66

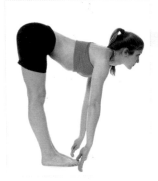

4 Ardha Uttanasana

page 66

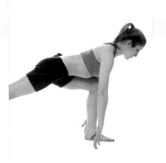

5 High Lunge

page 54

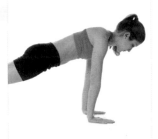

6 Plank Pose

page 128

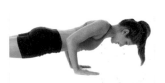

7 Chaturanga Dandasana

page 128

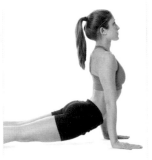

8 Urdhva Mukha Svanasana

page 84

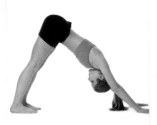

9 Adho Mukha Svanasana

page 22

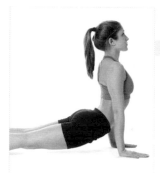

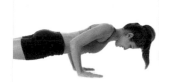

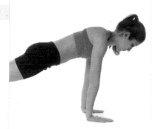

10 Urdhva Mukha Svanasana
page 84

11 Chaturanga Dandasana
page 128

12 Plank Pose
page 128

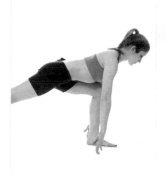

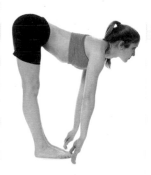

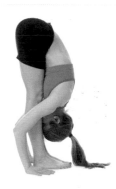

13 High Lunge
page 54

14 Ardha Uttanasana
page 66

15 Uttanasana
page 66

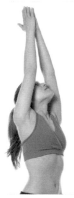

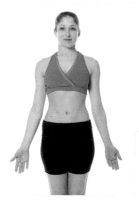

16 Urdhva Hastasana
page 24

17 Tadasana
page 30

SURYA NAMASKARA B

This alternate version of the Sun Salutation makes
an invigorating change to your morning yoga practice.

(Sun Salutation B)

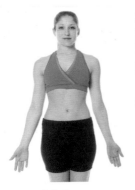

1 Tadasana

page 30

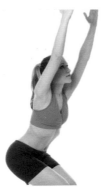

2 Utkatasana

page 34

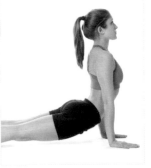

3 Uttanasana

page 66

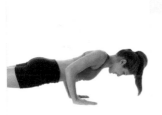

4 Chaturanga Dandasana

page 128

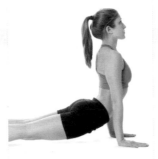

5 Urdhva Mukha Svanasana

page 84

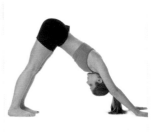

6 Adho Mukha Svanasana

page 22

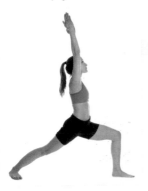

7 Virabhadrasana I

page 48

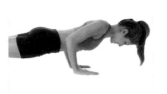

8 Chaturanga Dandasana

page 128

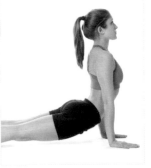

9 Urdhva Mukha Svanasana

page 84

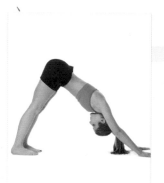

10 Adho Mukha Svanasana
page 22

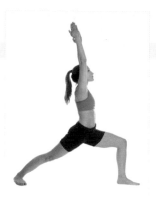

11 Virabhadrasana I
page 48

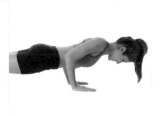

12 Chaturanga Dandasana
page 128

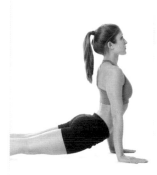

13 Urdhva Mukha Svanasana
page 84

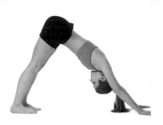

14 Adho Mukha Svanasana
page 22

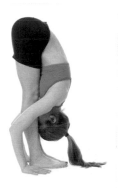

15 Uttanasana
page 66

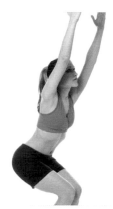

16 Utkatasana
page 34

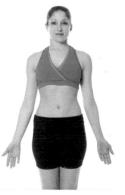

17 Tadasana
page 30

BEGINNER YOGA FLOW

Created for yoga novices, this yoga flow will take you through a variety of asana types, allowing you to establish a rhythmic flow as you begin your yoga practice.

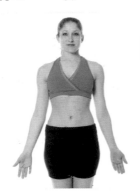

1 Tadasana

page 30

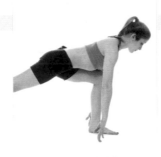

2 High Lunge

page 54

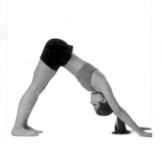

3 Adho Mukha Svanasana

page 22

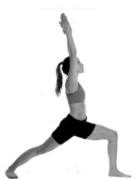

4 Virabhadrasana I

page 48

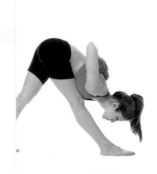

5 Parsvottanasana

page 76

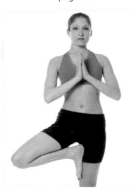

6 Virasana

page 21

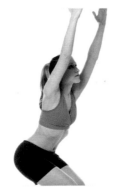

7 Utkatasana

page 34

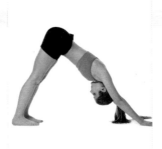

8 Adho Mukha Svanasana

page 22

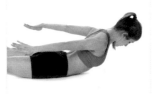

9 Salabhasana

page 86

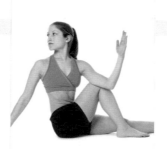

10 Paripurna Navasana
page 120

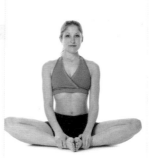

11 Marichyasana III
page 108

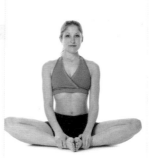

12 Baddha Konasana
page 68

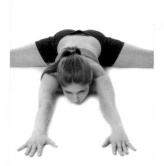

13 Upavistha Konasana
page 74

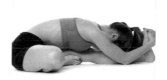

14 Janu Sirsasana
page 70

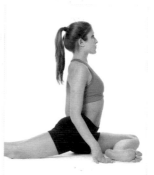

15 Eka Pada Rajakapotasana
page 102

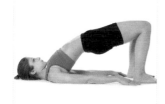

16 Setu Bandhasana
page 90

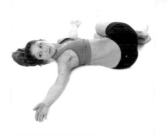

17 Jathara Parivartanasana
page 112

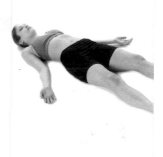

18 Savasana
page 27

INTERMEDIATE YOGA FLOW

This flow takes yoga practitioners with a bit of experience through a varied
sequence that includes all categories of asanas, from standing to balancing poses.

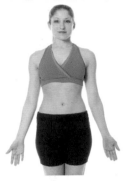

1 Tadasana

page 30

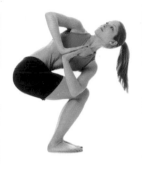

2 Parivrtta Utkatasana

page 36

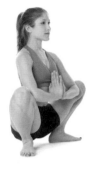

3 Malasana

page 38

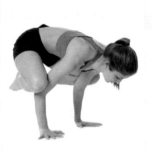

4 Bakasana

page 140

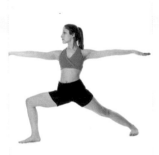

5 Virabhadrasana II

page 50

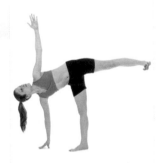

6 Ardha Chandrasana

page 58

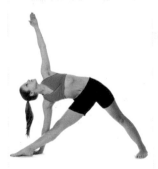

7 Trikonasana

page 42

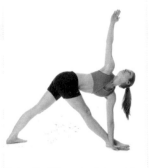

8 Parivrtta Trikonasana

page 60

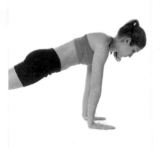

9 Plank Pose

page 128

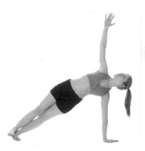

10 Vasisthasana
page 130

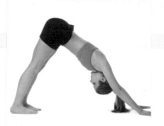

11 Adho Mukha Svanasana
page 22

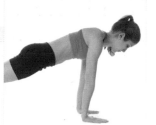

12 Plank Pose
page 128

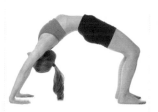

13 Urdhva Dhanurasana
page 98

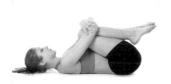

14 Apanasana
page 26

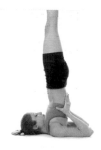

15 Salamba Sarvangasana
page 136

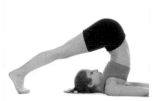

16 Halasana
page 134

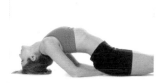

17 Matsyasana
page 88

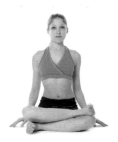

18 Agnistambhasana
page 20

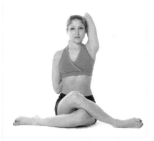

19 Gomukhasana
page 118

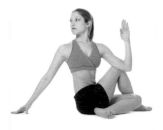

20 Ardha Matsyendrasana
page 116

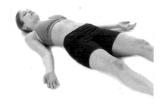

21 Savasana
page 27

ADVANCED YOGA FLOW

For the experienced practitioner who has gained strength and flexibility through dedicated practice, this flow challenges you with a variety of advanced asanas.

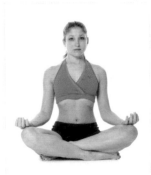

1 Sukhasana
page 18

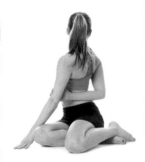

2 Bharadvajasana I
page 110

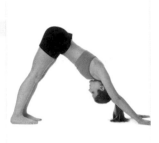

3 Adho Mukha Svanasana
page 22

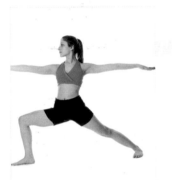

4 Virabhadrasana II
page 50

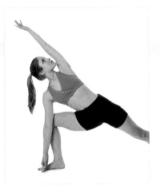

5 Utthita Parsvakonasana
page 44

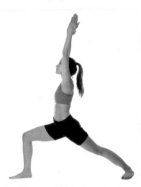

6 Virabhadrasana I
page 48

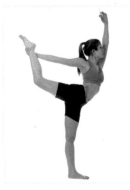

7 Natarajasana
page 104

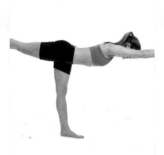

8 Virabhadrasana III
page 52

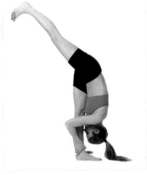

9 Urdhva Prasarita Eka Padasana
page 62

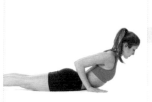

10 Bhujangasana
page 82

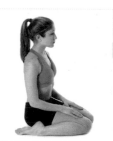

11 Virasana
page 21

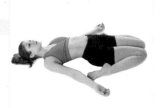

12 Supta Virasana
page 92

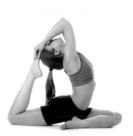

13 Eka Pada Rajakapotasana
page 102

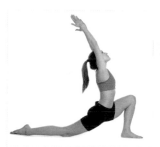

14 Anjaneyasana
page 46

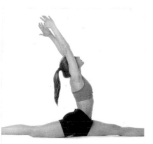

15 Hanumanasana
124

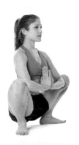

16 Malasana
page 38

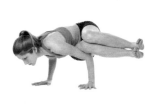

17 Parsva Bakasana
page 142

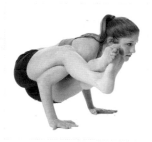

18 Astavakrasana
page 144

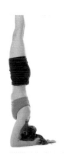

19 Salamba Sirsasana
page 138

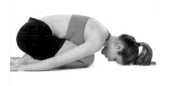

20 Balasana
page 25

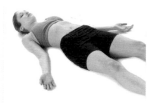

21 Savasana
page 27

INDEX OF ENGLISH NAMES

CREDITS

Created by Lisa Purcell Editorial & Design for Moseley Road, Inc.

Moseley Road Inc.
123 Main Street
Irvington, New York 10533

President: Sean Moore
Production director: Adam Moore
Project art and editorial director: Lisa Purcell

Photographer: Jonathan Conklin Photography, Inc.

Model: Goldie Karpel Oren

Retoucher: Mayoca Design

Illustrator: Hector Aiza/3DLabz

Full-body illustrations and insets: Linda Bucklin/Shutterstock.com

ABOUT THE AUTHORS

A retired gymnast, Amy Auman found her way into Yoga and Pilates after suffering from a back injury. Primarily practiced in Bikram and Vinyasa, she has since regained her strength, flexibility, and focus. Amy earned her BFA from Washington University in St. Louis. She now works as a consultant, designer, and adjunct lecturer based in St. Louis, Missouri.

Lisa Purcell is a New York City book designer, editor, and writer. A graduate of Princeton University, she specializes in health and fitness books.